Delirium in Critical Care

Second Edition

CORE CRITICAL CARE

Series Editor
Dr Alain Vuylsteke
Papworth Hospital
Cambridge, UK

Assistant Editor
Mrs Jo-anne Fowles
Papworth Hospital
Cambridge, UK

Other titles in the series
Intra-Abdominal Hypertension
Manu Malbrain and Jan De Waele
ISBN 9780521149396

Clinical Information Systems in Critical Care
Cecily Morrison, Matthew R. Jones and Julie Bracken
ISBN 9780521156745

Forthcoming titles in the series
Renal Replacement Therapy in Critical Care
Patrick Honoré and Oliver Joannes-Boyau
ISBN 9780521145404

ECMO in the Adult Patient
Alain Combes and Giles Peek
ISBN 9781107681248

Delirium in critical care

Second Edition

Valerie J. Page, MD
Consultant in Critical Care
Watford General Hospital
Watford, UK

E. Wesley Ely, MD, MPH
Professor of Medicine
Vanderbilt University School of Medicine and
Vanderbilt University Medical Center
Nashville, TN, USA

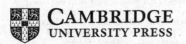

CAMBRIDGE
UNIVERSITY PRESS

CAMBRIDGE
UNIVERSITY PRESS

University Printing House, Cambridge CB2 8BS, United Kingdom

One Liberty Plaza, 20th Floor, New York, NY 10006, USA

477 Williamstown Road, Port Melbourne, VIC 3207, Australia

314-321, 3rd Floor, Plot 3, Splendor Forum, Jasola District Centre, New Delhi - 110025, India

79 Anson Road, #06-04/06, Singapore 079906

Cambridge University Press is part of the University of Cambridge.

It furthers the University's mission by disseminating knowledge in the pursuit of
education, learning and research at the highest international levels of excellence.

www.cambridge.org
Information on this title: www.cambridge.org/9781107433656

First published 2011
Second Edition 2015
3rd printing 2018

A catalogue record for this publication is available from the British Library

Library of Congress Cataloging in Publication data
Page, Valerie J., 1959- author.
Delirium in critical care / Valerie J., Page, E. Wesley Ely. – Second edition.
     p. ; cm. – (Core critical care)
Includes bibliographical references and index.
ISBN 978-1-107-43365-6 (Paperback)
I. Ely, E. Wesley, author.   II. Title.   III. Series: Core critical care.
[DNLM: 1. Critical Care.   2. Delirium. WL 340]
RC520.7
616.02´8–dc23   2014010873

ISBN 978-1-107-43365-6 Paperback

....

Every effort has been made in preparing this book to provide accurate and
up-to-date information which is in accord with accepted standards and practice
at the time of publication. Although case histories are drawn from actual cases,
every effort has been made to disguise the identities of the individuals involved.
Nevertheless, the authors, editors and publishers can make no warranties that the
information contained herein is totally free from error, not least because clinical
standards are constantly changing through research and regulation. The authors,
editors and publishers therefore disclaim all liability for direct or consequential
damages resulting from the use of material contained in this book. Readers
are strongly advised to pay careful attention to information provided by the
manufacturer of any drugs or equipment that they plan to use.

We dedicate this book to our fathers,
both of whom suffered delirium during critical illness.

CONTENTS

FOREWORD TO THE FIRST EDITION

The identification of delirium as an important entity in acutely
and critically ill patients has been one of major advances in
intensive care over the last decade. There is increasing
recognition that the condition has an important impact on
morbidity, health economics and patient outcome, not just in
critical care, but also in the perioperative period, during acute
medical illness, and at the end of life. However, there has also
been a realization that the condition is under diagnosed, and
that its prevention and treatment are frequently neglected.
Given this context, this book is a welcome resource for
clinicians who are involved in treating patients who are at risk
of delirium or require treatment for the condition. The authors
are practising clinicians with complementary backgrounds
in critical care. Professor Wesley Ely is perhaps the best
recognized expert in this field worldwide, whose publications
have put delirium on the critical care agenda. Dr Valerie
Page runs a busy general intensive care unit and brings her
experience of everyday critical care to the problem, along
with knowledge of the background literature. While this book
does provide some information on the clinical science and
neurobiology underpinning the condition, this is not its main
attraction, and there is a refreshing candor about the

substantial and large lacunae in knowledge about delirium. Its great strength lies in its practicality, and in the robust clinical sense that it displays in guiding the practising ICU doctor or nurse through the process of detecting, classifying, quantifying, preventing and treating delirium. The resource that it provides should make individual clinicians and ICU teams more aware of the condition, and in doing this, could help improve patient outcomes.

David K. Menon
Professor of Anaesthesia,
University of Cambridge, UK

FOREWORD TO THE SECOND EDITION

As authors Valerie Page and Wes Ely remind us in their introduction of Chapter 1, delirium is an 'an acute episode of brain failure'. As with acute failures of other organs, delirium is 'common ... dangerous ... even life-threatening'. Yet delirium has lagged behind the other major organ failure syndromes in its status in routine clinical practice. This book is an important resource in addressing this gap through providing a highly user-friendly distillate of the best in clinical practice and research.

Valerie Page and Wes Ely are practising clinicians and researchers. Alongside her clinical work as an intensivist in a busy general hospital in Watford, Dr Page has contributed several important trials to the field. She also founded and edits *Annals of Delirium*, the newsletter of the European Delirium Association, and is an active member of the Association's board. Professor Ely and his team at Vanderbilt University have produced the world's largest body of globally influential studies on delirium care in the ICU. Professor Ely is also an exceptionally energetic advocate for the well-being of patients with delirium through his multiple international lectures and site visits, and his support of the work of the American Delirium Society.

This book is comprehensive and all key areas are covered. Two highlights to mention here are detection, and the appropriate use of drugs. Though it is axiomatic that optimal care cannot be provided without a diagnosis, gross underdetection of delirium is a persisting challenge in clinical practice. The authors tackle both the *why* and the *how* of detection. Evidence confirming the high prevalence of ICU delirium is summarized, and major findings from the new BRAIN-ICU study on outcomes of ICU delirium from Professor Ely's team are described. This study shows that increased duration of delirium predicts worse cognitive outcomes 3 and 12 months after the episode of delirium, with the implication that detection and then good care has the potential to make a difference in the long term. Another compelling *why* is patient distress, and this is richly illustrated through many case histories. The authors also provide readers with valuable and pragmatic information on the *how*. They discuss the new diagnostic criteria for delirium (DSM-5, published in May 2013), providing clear guidance on interpretation of these new criteria. They also offer the reader valuable detail on the use of the two major clinical rating scales used to detect and monitor delirium in the ICU, the Confusion Assessment Method for the ICU (CAM-ICU) and the Intensive Care Delirium Screening Checklist (ICDSC). The book also gives substantial coverage of the current state of the art in the appropriate use of drugs in delirium treatment alongside the differential risks of sedatives and other drugs in causing delirium. New findings showing relative benefits of dexmedetomidine over benzodiazepines, the likely lack of efficacy of haloperidol, and others are discussed. Other notable new content in the second edition relates to new methods of prediction of delirium risk, the role of the ICU environment in modifying delirium risk and the patient experience, and novel evidence on practical and effective methods of delirium prevention in the ICU.

In summary, this second edition builds upon the great success of the first. The content is grounded in both the recent scientific evidence as well as hands-on clinical knowledge. Busy clinicians in the ICU will find no better concise and yet wide-ranging guide to this challenging area of medicine.

Alasdair M. J. MacLullich

Professor of Geriatric Medicine,

Edinburgh Delirium Research Group,

University of Edinburgh, and

President of the European Delirium Association

REFERENCES

American Psychiatric Association. Neurocognitive disorders. *Diagnostic and Statistical Manual of Mental Disorders*, 5th edn, DSM-V. Arlington, VA, American Psychiatric Publishing. 2013; 591–602.

DELIRIUM, A PATIENT TESTIMONY

As birthdays go, this one was absolute rubbish. It was 8 o'clock on a May evening in 2007, and where I should have been enjoying an evening out with my husband and friends, here I was sitting in A & E with a broken nose, the result of the most mundane of domestic accidents – falling over some washing while I was completely sober.

Two weeks later I was summoned for day surgery to sort the nose out. My conversation with a porter about the next day's FA Cup final, while making my way down to theatre, is the last memory I have before being plunged into the most terrifying experience of my life.

The next occasion when I had any perception of time was 12 days later, when I found myself being stared at by two middle-aged men in dark suits and bright ties. One was busily explaining to me that I was in the Intensive Care Unit and that I was quite safe.

However, I knew better. I knew they were lying. For me, the reason I was in a bed, on a ventilator, hardly able to move, was that I had been drugged and kidnapped. It had all started in Portugal; at least I thought it was Portugal, where I'd been abducted. At some point I'd managed to escape but was re-captured and taken to a hospital, a few miles from my home.

I knew that I must have done something wrong, to be held with no hope of escape, but I had no idea what it was. I'd tried on several occasions to pull the tube out of my mouth, but had always been instantly plunged back into darkness.

It never crossed my mind that there might have been a medical reason for my predicament, and I had no knowledge that severe aspiration pneumonia following my routine surgery had landed me in ICU and was putting my family through hell.

What I did know with certainty though was that I would die. One particular doctor would visit me every time I started to wake. He always wore the same clothes and would always speak slowly and deliberately. 'You've been dying to know what that sign on the wall says, haven't you?', he asked one day. He was right; I had wondered what it said but the problem was I could see two of everything and objects and people were frequently blurred so I hadn't been able to read it. 'I'll tell you what it says' he continued. 'It says "moron". We put it there so every time you open your eyes it's the first thing you see; so that for every minute of every day you know exactly what you are. Unfortunately I'm not allowed to turn your ventilator off, but I want you out of here, and you will leave soon, in a body bag. You're not going to live, but just remember every time you open your eyes you will see exactly what we think of you – moron'.

From then on, that sign was the only thing I could see that wasn't blurred.

The rest of my stay in ICU was filled with more incidents of despair, humiliation and terror. I saw a patient stabbed to death by his wife, and two people committing suicide. I witnessed arguments, in my mind all caused by me, and the pain I felt as my lungs started to recover was all part of a plan to give me pain-inducing drugs – in fact I had seen doctors laughing about it.

The day after I was extubated I found myself in the High Dependency Unit, where the sheer terror of the execution attempts began. Initially I thought I was in the morgue as I was lying flat and was extremely cold. There was a plain clothes policeman watching me because I'd witnessed a murder on ICU. Someone spoke to me 'I can control your mind' they said, and then proceeded to demonstrate they had power over me by causing me pain and by interrupting my supply of oxygen at will.

The following morning a tall and distinguished looking man sat down and explained to me that I had Pershing's disease. This was a rare congenital heart condition that can lie dormant for many years. Once a sufferer shows symptoms, however, their life expectancy is less than a year. In my mind I might as well just die where I was, and the doctor encouraged me to do exactly that. Pershing's disease of course, does not exist, but just like everything else that happened to me, the hallucination I had where it was explained was so convincing that I was still trying to find evidence of its existence weeks later.

I was put into a side room in the High Dependency Unit, allegedly for infection control, but I knew it was for my execution. I'd heard the nurses talk about CTO, which was a Compulsory Termination Order, and one had been issued for me. As the blinds were pulled down over the room's windows and door, smoke appeared through every vent. A voice told me it was cyanide and I would die more quickly if I relaxed and *inhaled it. I watched it creep closer, paralysed with terror, and all I could think about was that I would never see my family again.*

Having somehow survived, the execution attempts continued. They included suffocation, poisoning, drug overdoses and being forced to hold my breath until four lights went out on my monitor. By the time I moved down to a respiratory ward I had given up trying to convince my family that the hospital staff were trying to kill me. I still had no idea of what was wrong with me, and when my husband explained, I was sure that all my problems had been induced and had not simply happened. It was then that I decided to keep quiet about my views as no one believed me or was prepared to help me, so I planned my escape alone. By this time I could take some of my medications orally, so this gave me some element of control, as I would wait until the nurse left the room, then would throw the pills containing poison into the medical waste. I ate nothing at mealtimes, but instead stole pieces of cutlery that would help me prise my window open. I was utterly oblivious to the fact that I was four floors up. The hallucinations had stopped by now but were replace by paranoia and deviousness. The day I planned to leave via the window was the day I was discharged. That might seem lucky, but I spent the next few months wishing that I had died that day.

My physical recovery once I was home moved forward very quickly, but inside I was in meltdown. I couldn't tell anyone how I really felt – my family and friends had been through so much already. My delirium and its consequences caused me to believe that I was still being poisoned, even after leaving hospital, so I stopped taking my medication.

*What do I wish had been different for me? Well, when
I received a copy of my medical notes following a suggestion that
it would help me to make some sense of what had happened,
I read through the hundreds of pages that comprised a file
6 inches thick. Only once did I find a relevant reference. It was
one about me being severely paranoid, and that note was made
by a physiotherapist. Although I have no doubts whatsoever that
the care I received was of the highest order, I still feel today that
my delirium was seen as an acceptable side effect of my illness
and treatment. Months later, during my ICU follow-up
appointment, they were not at all surprised that I had suffered
prolonged and extreme delirium; in fact they appeared to know
I had. To them it was 'normal'. To me it was anything but.*

*Two years have now passed since my experience of delirium.
In that time I've been able to make sense of at least some of
what happened to me. My mother reminded me that my belief
I'd been kidnapped could well have been my brain confusing my
situation with something that had been constantly in the news.
Unfortunately, I'd shared my birthday, the day of my accident,
with the day that Madeleine McCann was taken from her family's
holiday apartment in Portugal, and the tragedy had been at the
top of every news bulletin leading up to the day of my surgery.*

*I know too that my almost total lack of memory for the
routine events you would expect to experience on a hospital
ward, and which would have reassured me about where I was
and what was happening, stopped me from challenging my
warped and terrifying perception of the world.*

*Whatever the future holds though, I'm never doing the
washing on my birthday again.*

Chapter 1

What is delirium in critical care?

Introduction

Imagine you are caring for a critically ill patient admitted with severe community-acquired pneumonia. Unfortunately, this evolves rapidly with severe sepsis that results in both cardiovascular and respiratory failure. You know the patient has haemodynamic failure because you are monitoring the blood pressure and heart rate. You know the patient has respiratory failure because you are monitoring the respiratory rate and the oxygen saturation. You treat the patient with antibiotics, ventilatory support, fluids and inotropes.

He gets better, a job well done.

But what about the brain?

Just like the other organs, the brain can acutely fail in critical illness. An acute episode of brain failure is recognized as delirium. Delirium is an acute organ failure, and can happen in critical care, the general ward or the community at large. It is common; it is dangerous, even life-threatening. It is all the more dangerous because we know little about it. Its importance has been underestimated in the critically ill patient. The delirious patient is in an acute confusional state with a fluctuating altered mental status, inattention, an altered level of consciousness, disorganized thinking and often will have hallucinations. The delirium is triggered by an acute medical event, related to drugs or illness.

We therefore need to monitor the brain!

We monitor the patient's organs so we will know how they are functioning and when they are failing. If we do not monitor the brain how will we know if it fails?

But how can we do so?

Any critically ill patient who responds to a verbal stimulus such as calling their name can be screened for delirium in less than 2 minutes whether intubated or not, on or off sedation.

Delirium is a clinical syndrome and is diagnosed at the bedside, but it is not always easy to recognize. The majority of delirious patients are not agitated, pulling at lines and tubes, climbing out of bed; in fact they are lethargic and sleepy. If you want to know if your patient's brain is healthy you will need to check for function.

Fortunately this is quick and easy.

Does it affect the outcome?

Back to our patient with respiratory failure, 4 months later. He attends the follow-up clinic with his wife. His wife reports that he can't concentrate; he keeps forgetting friend's names, even those he has known for years. He can't remember where he has left things; all his vitality seems to have gone. Cardiovascular and respiratory functions are back to normal. Heart and lungs cured, brain irreversibly damaged...

Recognizing delirium allows initiation of treatment

Delirium is associated with serious adverse outcomes including death; your delirious patient is a medical emergency.

History

One syndrome, delirium, has been given many names. While Hippocrates is credited with the first description of delirium even he used about 16 different words! Amongst them were *phrenitis* (or frenzy) and *lethargus* and he described patients that would oscillate between the two delirious states. In today's terminology these are now called hyperactive, hypoactive and mixed motoric subtypes. Hippocrates also noted that patients were often fidgety, plucking at the air and at their bedclothes. Clinical signs observed nearly 2500 years ago are still present today – just the bedclothes are different!

The word delirium appears for the first time in *De Medicina*. This document is what is left of a large encyclopaedia compiled by Celsus, a Roman living under the reign of Tiberius (around AD 1). It was only rediscovered around 1480 in Milan. *De Medicina* was soon widely published, and

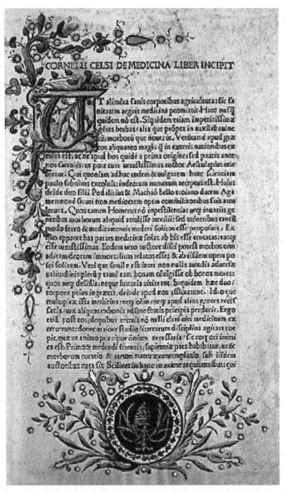

Figure 1.1 Aulus Cornelius Celsus, *De Medicina*, 1478, Florentine.
Courtesy of the Historical Medical Library of The College of
Physicians of Philadelphia.

became one of the most important ancient sources for Renaissance medicine. Celsus used the word delirium to describe mental disorders during fever or head trauma. He reported that wine could be used as part of the treatment when not associated with fever (recognizing alcohol dependence as a possible cause of delirium). The word delirium derives from the Latin *deliro–delirare* that literally means going off track, a sharp description of a wandering brain!

The historian Procopius comes next and has left us a precise description of delirium during the bubonic plague when reporting about a possible epidemic in Constantinople in AD 542:

For there ensued with some a deep coma, with others a violent delirium, and in either case they suffered the characteristic symptoms of the disease. For those who were under the spell of coma forgot all those who were familiar to them and seemed to lie sleeping constantly ... those who were seized with delirium suffered from insomnia and were victims of a distorted imagination.

It was not until the early 1800s that Greiner suggested that clouding of consciousness was the main pathogenic feature of delirium. This led Hughlings Jackson to define consciousness at the turn of the last century, as one function of the central nervous system that could be disturbed by different agents leading to positive and negative signs of disturbance.

Engel and Romano were the first to show that the reduction in the level of consciousness seen in delirious patients could be correlated to electroencephalogram (EEG) activity. This 'unifying' interpretation was based on psychopathological characteristics and concluded that the disturbance in consciousness results in the failure of different cognitive tasks, fluctuating levels of awareness, psychomotor hyper- or hypoactivity, agitation or lethargy. In 1959 they complained that clinicians were ill-equipped to recognize delirium and that more should be done to train them to recognize the problem. They declared that a physician's concerns are to 'protect the functional integrity of the heart, liver and kidneys of his patient but has not learnt to have similar regard for the functional integrity of the brain'.

Dr Lipowski, a Polish-born, Irish-trained psychiatrist who settled in North America, proposed a definition of delirium in 1990 that has been very influential in the most recent psychiatric classifications. Delirium is 'a transient, global disorder of cognition, consciousness and attention regardless of the level of consciousness (awareness) or psychomotor activity that a given patient exhibits which may often change from one extreme to another in the course of a single day'; or a 'transient organic mental syndrome of acute onset, characterized by global impairment of cognitive functions, a reduced level of consciousness, attentional abnormalities, increased or decreased psychomotor activity and disordered sleep–wake cycle' (adapted from Lipowski [1]).

Other recent key players include Dr Sharon Inouye, who developed the Confusion Assessment Method, and Dr Paula Trzepacz working in key areas of phenomenology and neuropathogenesis.

Throughout history delirium has been described as a serious clinical condition with a poor prognosis. Hippocrates noted 'cases of silent delirium, with restlessness, a changing gaze . . . are likely to prove fatal'. Also delirium associated with gnashing meant almost certain death. Philip Barrough in 1593 noted that it is an incurable and deadly condition in most cases. Importantly he added that, in the rare cases where it did resolve, it might be followed by memory loss and an inability to reason.

Classification

In the 1970s the American Psychiatric Association developed the *Diagnostic and Statistical Manual of Mental Disorders*, better known as DSM, to provide diagnostic criteria for mental disorders. Updated versions have been published, and these will continue to evolve as new data from research and clinical experience emerge. The latest is the DSM-5 in which delirium and all subtypes of dementia are classified under cognitive disorders, the unifying feature being a primary clinical deficit in cognitive function, acquired rather than developmental.

The alternative *International Classification of Diseases* (ICD) by the World Health Organization (WHO) has a broader remit as the international standard diagnostic classification for all general epidemiological use, many health management purposes and clinical use. It is now at its tenth revision (ICD-10). The next one, ICD-11, is due around 2016.

Regarding delirium the ICD-10 is overall similar to the DSM-5. Both are classifications of mental disorders based on diagnostic criteria, i.e. history, examination and clinical tests, and were first compiled from a need to bring order to the

Table 1.1 Diagnostic criteria for delirium

1. Disturbance of consciousness: Reduced clarity of awareness of the environment with reduced ability to focus, sustain or shift attention
2. A change in cognition: Memory deficit, disorientation, language disturbance or the development of a perceptual disturbance that is not better accounted for by a pre-existing, established or evolving dementia
3. Develops over a short period of time and fluctuates: Usually hours to days. Tends to fluctuate during the course of the day
4. There is evidence that the disturbance is caused by the direct physiological consequences of a general medical condition. History, physical examination or laboratory finding
5. Patient is not in a severely reduced level of arousal equivalent to being comatose

chaotic psychiatric terminology, a result of the different theoretical models and 'schools' of thought that have existed for a long period.

Medical literature on delirium almost always quote DSM-IV criteria as a reference standard for the diagnosis. Shortly before the publication of DSM-5, the US National Institute of Mental Health made a decision to move away from clinical checklist DSM criteria, to a research framework they have developed (Research Domain Criteria). The rationale is to look beyond symptoms alone and collect genetic, imaging, physiological and cognitive data.

DSM-5 criteria

The DSM-5, the fifth edition, was published in May 2013. There are five diagnostic criteria, against four in the fourth edition.

Starting with a disturbance of attention, 'i.e. to direct, focus, sustain or shift attention' (or more simply, inattention), which develops within a short time and fluctuates. This is combined with an additional disturbance of cognition, e.g. memory loss, disorientation, language disturbance; or a perceptual disturbance, such as hallucinations or delusional thoughts, not known to be caused by another cognitive disorder such as established or developing dementia. Delirium cannot be established as present in a patient with a severely reduced level of arousal, i.e. comatose. While in practice hallucinations are relatively common in delirium they are not needed for the diagnosis. Finally there must be clinical evidence that there is a medical cause or causes, either illness, toxin or drug related.

After establishing that a patient fulfils these criteria the DSM classifies delirium into groups dependent on the presumed cause and specifies it as substance intoxication or withdrawal, medication induced, due to another medical condition – the name of which should be noted – or delirium due to multiple aetiologies, which is the section most likely to apply to critically ill patients. Further useful information is whether the delirium is acute, i.e. lasting days, or persistent, and hyperactive, hypoactive or mixed (see Chapter 3).

New to DSM-5, so absent from DSM-IV, is the criterion that the disturbances of attention and change in cognition should not be present in a patient with severely reduced level of arousal 'such as coma'. Importantly, the accompanying text notes that some patients with a reduced level of arousal, as is typical in delirium, may only show minimal responses such that they are incapable of engaging with assessment of attention. DSM-5 determines that this inability to engage is severe inattention, which, combined with the low-arousal state, indicates the patient has delirium. This is seen in critically ill patients who, while they will open their eyes, do not squeeze your hand on request at all for assessment of delirium (see Chapter 7).

It is important to note that whilst guidance is given regarding differentiation of delirium from dementia, patients with dementia are particularly vulnerable to delirium, presenting with delirium superimposed on top of dementia.

Terminology in critical care

In 1990, over 30 terms used to refer to delirium were identified in the medical literature (Figure 1.2). It is tempting to bring back terms such as 'subacute befuddlement' or maybe 'dysergastic reaction' but of course it is unlikely this would lead to intensivists taking delirium more seriously. Critical care lent its name to ICU psychosis and ICU syndrome, often to allow the delirium to be dismissed as an expected and inconsequential complication of critical illness. Other names, such as septic encephalopathy, hepatic encephalopathy, toxic confusional state, acute confusional state, metabolic encephalopathy or acute brain syndrome, highlight how important the syndrome is *in these situations*. But no delirium can be supposed benign or self-limiting.

The failure to standardize terminology may be one reason why delirium has not been given to date the scientific consideration it deserves, even if the multiplicity of terms and

Table 1.2 Broad division of delirium as per DSM-5 classification

Name	Comments
General medical condition	Specific cause does not need to be identified if evidence for medical disorder present
Substance-induced	Intoxication or withdrawal
Multiple aetiologies	More than one cause identified
Not otherwise specified	Diagnostic criteria present, no cause identified

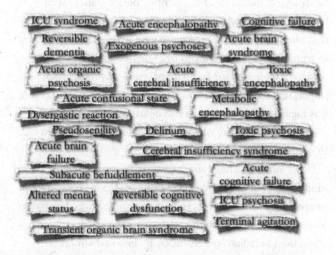

Figure 1.2 Non-exhaustive list of some of the numerous terms used to refer to delirium.

descriptions suggests a high prevalence. Maybe the many different names were attempts over the years to make clinicians take it seriously (familiarity breeds contempt).

On the other hand perhaps it is a reflection of how widespread delirium is throughout different patient populations in whom it keeps being 'rediscovered'.

Acute and fluctuating disturbances of consciousness and cognition, and inattention are the common features in all patients with delirium, whatever the cause.

Identifying the cause is definitely important to guide prevention, management and therapy but it is unknown whether the trigger itself is relevant to the patient's neurological outcomes. For example, does a patient who became delirious while being ventilated for acute respiratory distress syndrome (ARDS) end up with worse delirium-related outcomes than a patient who became delirious with a simple urinary tract infection? Is a patient's genetic profile more important? For these reasons, and in accordance with DSM-5, it is logical and important to use delirium as the standard name, with the cause, when known, noted – e.g. delirium due to sepsis.

Other languages have similar issues. For example the medical term in Italian that corresponds to Lipowski's definition of acute confusional state is *stato confusionale acuto*. The Italian word *delirio* in medical terminology means delusion although when used in Italian lay vocabulary is close to delirium.

In France delirium is almost always shorthand for delirium tremens – i.e. associated with alcohol withdrawal. They use *confusion mentale* for delirium as described in DSM-IV.

The only conditions all agree on are coma/*koma* and delirium tremens.

To align terminology between countries is important, hence the WHO released in 1993 diagnostic criteria for clinical research, the ICD-10-DR. This intends to help clinical researchers to communicate and also to align ICD-10 and DSM. The current six criteria concerning delirium relate to consciousness and cognition with fluctuation, disturbance of sleep pattern and evidence of a clinical cause.

Key points

- Delirium indicates an acute organ failure.
- Delirium has always been known to be associated with poor outcomes.
- Standard diagnostic criteria for delirium are in the DSM-5 and the ICD-10.
- There are a number of clinical terms in use to describe delirium including ICU psychosis and acute confusional state. All delirium, all serious.

FURTHER READING

A podcast overview by Dr Valerie Page. http://letsrespect.co.uk/resources/podcasts/.

Adamis D *et al.* A brief review of the history of delirium as a mental disorder. *History of Psychiatry* 2007; 18: 459–69.

American Psychiatric Association. Neurocognitive disorders. *Diagnostic and Statistical Manual of Mental Disorders*, 5th edn, DSM-5. Arlington, VA, American Psychiatric Publishing. 2013; 591–602.

Chapter 2

How common is delirium in critical care?

The numbers game

Delirium has a wide diversity of names and multiple possible causes (see Chapter 1). It can clinically be seen as stupor, agitation or both. Theories about its pathophysiology abound – and all of them may prove correct. The criteria used to diagnose delirium evolve continuously and the literature and research relating to delirium are dogged by ambiguity. As a result, the prevalence will depend on case mix, duration of screening and screening tool used.

The overall picture

It is known that overall 1:6 patients will be delirious in any general hospital ward, with the greatest incidence found in intensive care (1:5 in high dependency patients and up to 4:5 in ventilated patients). Some clinicians believe that delirium is merely a reflection of how critically ill the patient is rather than being of any importance in itself. But the evidence clearly demonstrates that delirium is associated with seriously adverse outcomes, independent of the severity of the patient's illness.

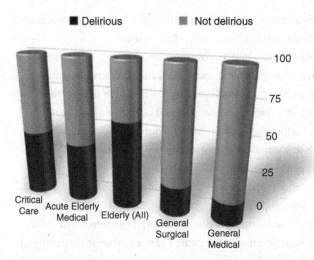

Figure 2.1 **Proportion of patients delirious in a general hospital at any one time.**

Different clinical areas will have a different number of patients affected, with an incidence of around 2:5 in an acute geriatrics ward, and 3:5 in patients who have suffered a fractured neck of femur.

This means that on any given day in an acute general hospital of around 1000 beds, there will be more than 100 delirious patients!

Detecting delirium

Clinicians who have not used a delirium screening tool will fail to recognize it in a significant number of patients even if they are actively considering the diagnosis. Studies in elderly hospital patients demonstrate that clinicians do not recognize delirium in up to three out of four cases.

Sharon Inouye *et al.* compared in 2001 how nurses rated delirium in a non-ICU ward when using observations during routine clinical care without formal cognitive testing, with the rating of a researcher using formal cognitive assessment [2]. In addition, they interviewed the nurses seeking evidence of each individual feature of delirium (i.e. inattention, disorganized thinking, altered level of consciousness, disorientation, memory problems or inappropriate behaviour). The nurses identified delirium in less than 1:3 of patients marked as delirious by the researchers, but never marked a patient as delirious if the patient was not, showing a very good negative discriminatory assessment (have not) but a very poor positive discriminatory assessment (have). Importantly, the nurses identified inattention only 15% of the time when this feature was present. This is noteworthy as it is an essential feature of delirium and is looked for in most general screening tools. Four independent risk factors leading to under-recognition of delirium by nurses were identified: hypoactive delirium, age 80 years or older, vision impairment and dementia. Paradoxically, there was an increased risk of failing to identify delirium with an increasing number of risk factors being present.

This was in a hospital ward setting with the carers able to talk with the patients. It is not surprising that the risk of failure to recognize delirium in critical care is even higher with ventilated patients! This was proven by van Eijk *et al.* who conducted a similar study in critical care and showed a clinical

Table 2.1 A list of some of the most commonly used tests to diagnose delirium in the non-ICU setting

DSM-IV-TR
Cognitive Test for Delirium
Confusion Assessment Method
Delirium Detection Score
Delirium Index
Delirium Rating Scale-Revised-98
Delirium Severity Scale
Delirium Symptom Interview
Memorial Delirium Assessment Scale
Neecham Confusion Scale
Short Portable Mental Status Questionnaire

detection rate (based on medical staff impression) in less than 1:3 delirious patients [3].

There are a number of validated tests to diagnose delirium in non-ICU patients (Table 2.1) and seven that have been described to evaluate delirium in the ICU. Only four of these have been validated against the DSM-IV criteria and only two are useful in intubated patients. These screening tests are described in detail in Chapter 7.

Incidence or prevalence?

The variation in the incidence quoted in studies using screening tools can be in part explained by the case mix and recruitment criteria set. The incidences quoted in this book are based on the critical care validated tool (see Chapter 7) unless otherwise specified.

Prevalence includes the number of patients already delirious on admission, while incidence refers to the proportion of patients who develop delirium during their critical care stay.

The delirium status of many patients on admission is often not known as they are sedated (and to be fair is also not recorded in most studies). When both prevalence and incidence are given in elderly patients admitted to medical critical care, around 30% of patients are delirious on initial assessment and most clinicians will see patients regularly admitted to critical care in 'acute confusional state' – i.e. delirious.

CAM-ICU and ICDSC

The majority of studies quoting an incidence of ICU delirium use either the **C**onfusion **A**ssessment **M**ethod for the ICU (CAM-ICU) or the **I**ntensive **C**are **D**elirium **S**creening **C**hecklist (ICDSC), both of which were created in North America. Both

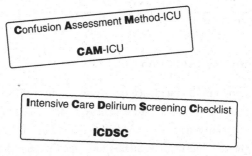

Figure 2.2 CAM-ICU and ICDSC abbreviations.

have since been used in other countries and the CAM-ICU has been translated into 20 languages. Both tests are detailed in Chapter 7.

The published incidence figures vary, seemingly depending on whether the ICDSC or the CAM-ICU is used. Both methods appear to be less effective than initially described, as is often the case when tests are used in routine practice rather than research. Profoundly sedated patients cannot be assessed using either test. A meta-analysis found that both tools are valid and useful to diagnose delirium in critically ill patients, but any screening tool will inevitably be imperfect, because of the difficulty in diagnosing delirium in any hospital patient. CAM-ICU and ICDSC have been endorsed by the American College of Critical Care Medicine as the most valid and reliable delirium monitoring tools available.

Tables 2.2 and 2.3 report values taken from various publications across several years and show a wide variation

Table 2.2 Incidence of delirium in the critically ill using ICDSC

Number of patients	Case mix	APACHE (mean)	Delirious
93	Mixed ICU	14	16%
198	Mixed ICU	15.2	19%
185	Mixed ICU 77% ventilated	19	45%
764	Mixed ICU 79% ventilated	17.9	31.8%
537	Mixed ICU 58% ventilated	18.6	35.2%

in the incidence. With regard to the ICDSC it was shown that level of consciousness did not discriminate well for delirium and in fact weakened the scale. In consequence, the level of consciousness in sedated patients and inattention in some patients are not used to diagnose delirium.

In contrast, inattention in the CAM-ICU is important whether the patient is on or off sedative drugs. The clinicians who use the CAM-ICU make the point that as the cause of delirium has not yet been shown to be important in terms of outcomes, it is still likely that the reduction in level of consciousness and inattention are important, even if apparently caused by sedation.

Conversely, the ICDSC includes hallucinations as a positive indicator for delirium, but these are not included in the CAM-ICU. There are patients who will screen as CAM-ICU negative who are quite clearly hallucinating. Clinically this may indicate subsyndromal rather than full-blown delirium although the CAM-ICU has not been validated to diagnose an intermediate state of brain dysfunction.

Despite the differences, both scores have been validated against the DSM-IV criteria and are established as good tools in critically ill patients. From published studies the pooled sensitivity of the ICDSC is 74% with a specificity of 82%. The CAM-ICU has a pooled sensitivity of 80% and a specificity of 96%. This means that 18% of patients who screen positive for delirium using the ICDSC, and 4% of those positive using CAM-ICU, would not be diagnosed as delirious if assessed thoroughly by a psychiatrist. Given the consistently high specificity of the CAM-ICU, there is ongoing work to increase the sensitivity of the test, particularly in non-intubated critically ill patients (see Chapter 7).

When examining the APACHE (the **A**cute **P**hysiology and **C**hronic **H**ealth **E**valuation score – higher the number, sicker the patient) scores in Tables 2.2 and 2.3, patients screened with CAM-ICU were sicker than patients screened with the ICDSC. It is now known that each increment in APACHE score increases the risk of delirium by around 5% and the difference in the reported incidence disappears when comparing patients with similar APACHE scores.

Expect a higher incidence of delirium in sicker patients!

Table 2.3 Incidence of delirium in the critically ill using CAM-ICU

Number of patients	Case mix	APACHE (mean)	Delirious
336	Medical ICU All ventilated	26	71%–74%
174	Surgical ICU including elective % ventilated unknown	25	41%
304	Medical ICU 54% ventilated	20–25	70%
614	Medical ICU 49% ventilated	20	72% when > 65 years old 57% if younger
114	Surgical ICU 49% ventilated	14.5	30% if > 65 years old
100	Surgical ICU All ventilated	24	73% surgical 67% trauma

The incidence in different critical care studies is also variable depending on the case mix of patients studied. For example, one CAM-ICU validation study was largely in patients with sepsis and/or acute respiratory distress syndrome (ARDS) while one study of the ICDSC used a significant number of patients who had undergone major vascular surgery. The incidence of delirium following aortic aneurysm surgery has been quoted at 33% – much lower than what is seen in ARDS/septic patients.

One of the recurring comments about the CAM-ICU is that it may miss delirium as it is a 'moment-in-time assessment'. CAM-ICU can miss delirium because of an inexperienced user of the instrument, or early/mild inattention requiring a longer test to detect. This is possible but intriguing given the higher incidence figures reported by units using the CAM-ICU.

Duration of delirium

The duration of delirium in intensive care ranges from 2 to 3 days in medical patients, 1 to 5 days after major trauma and up to 8 days in elderly surgical patients. In practice in ICU the duration lasts as least as long as the precipitating factor.

A 70-year-old male who underwent an elective gastrooesophagectomy developed delirium post-operatively. This was initially thought to be mainly due to the morphine he needed following the failure of his thoracic epidural to control pain. The delirium was difficult to manage as he was on amiodarone and his QTc increased to 500 msec when he was given haloperidol. The jejunostomy had not been used because of

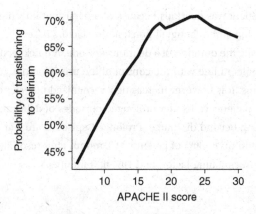

Figure 2.3 Probability of transitioning to delirium with increased
APACHE II score. Adapted with permission from Pandharipande *et al.*
Lorazepam is an independent risk factor for transitioning to delirium
in intensive care patients. *Anesthesiology* 2006; 104(1): 21–6.

*concerns over its integrity. He then developed sepsis and required
continuous veno-venous haemofiltration and vasopressor support. He
had two computed tomography scans, neither of which demonstrated
any abscess or other source of infection. Over the next 2 weeks he was
treated for a presumed respiratory infection, following which his organ
function improved and his blood tests returned to normal. Throughout
this time he seemed withdrawn and disinterested and intermittently
screened positive for delirium, using the CAM-ICU. It was thought he was
suffering from depression. After another week he showed signs of sepsis
again and was taken to theatre where a large infected collection
associated with his jejunostomy was drained. Postoperatively his mental
status improved and he was able to interact normally and positively with
friends and family.*

This patient was delirious because of a persistent infection. Identifying and treating all precipitating factors is key to modifying the duration of a delirious episode. A quick recovery is possible, in line with the control of the precipitating problems. It is however increasingly recognized that some elderly patients can suffer prolonged episodes of delirium persisting beyond discharge. Prolonged episodes are still present in up to 30% of patients at 1 month after resolution of the precipitating factor, and 18% at 3 months.

Incidence in special patient groups

Cardiac surgery

The incidences recorded following cardiac surgery are very variable and range from 8% in beating-heart coronary artery bypass grafting (off-pump) surgery to 67% in patients undergoing valve replacement. The reason for a high incidence linked to the use of cardiopulmonary bypass is not totally elucidated. Numerous small emboli of whatever origin, the inflammatory response or changes in flows are all possible culprits.

Trauma

It has always been thought that trauma patients are likely to develop delirium due to the associated head injury and accompanying inflammatory response. Trauma patients will often need high doses of sedatives and analgesics for pain relief and effective ventilation. The reported incidence is between 35% and 67%. The risk of developing delirium is higher in patients with a lower initial Glasgow Coma Score, increased blood transfusions and higher injury score.

Palliative care

The earliest medical observations indicated delirium was a sign of impending death. It is indeed very common in patients with advanced cancer, with incidence as high as 81%. Terminal delirium, defined as delirium occurring within 6 hours before death, is as high as 88%. For more information on delirium at the end of life, jump now to Chapter 11.

Key points

- Delirium is a common feature in intensive care.
- Without a screening tool clinicians will miss around three quarter of cases.
- CAM-ICU and ICDSC are both valid tools to screen ICU patients for delirium.
- The reported incidence of delirium will vary according to the tools used to detect it and the population studied.
- Sicker patients are more likely to suffer from delirium, and delirium is an independent predictor of worse outcomes.
- Delirium itself represents a clinical worsening in the patient's state of illness.

FURTHER READING

www.icudelirium.co.uk.

Inouye SK. Delirium in older persons. *New England Journal of Medicine* 2006; 354: 1157–65.

van Eijk MM *et al.* Comparison of delirium assessment tools in a mixed intensive care unit. *Critical Care Medicine* 2009; 37: 1881–5.

Chapter 3

What does delirium look like in critical care?

Introduction

Delirium is not a description of behaviour. Delirium is a medical diagnosis of a syndrome with specific diagnostic features, and significant morbidity and mortality. The diagnosis is primarily clinical and based on careful bedside observation of key features. In 1874 Fothergill writing about delirium summed up '... each case differs somewhat from every other case and there are peculiarities in each and every one'. Not very helpful!

Delirium is often missed by clinicians even when they are looking for it. In one intensive care study doctors missed nearly three quarters of cases although the consultants were considerably better at detecting delirium than the residents [3]. In an aptly titled paper *Occurrence of delirium is severely underestimated in the ICU*, it was shown that nurses picked up only 35% of daily delirium [4]. Though this was poor, this was considerably better than doctors who only detected daily delirium 28% of the time!

So why can delirium be difficult to identify?

Delirium is difficult to spot because it is often quiet – the lethargic patient who is unable to maintain attention is suffering from hypoactive delirium.

Yes! Take note! … the majority of delirium does not present with agitation. On the contrary patients' brains wind down and they become drowsy and reluctant to move rather than the brains winding up and causing hyperactivity. Lipowski called delirium a disorder of wakefulness – too much or too little.

Motoric subtypes

Three clinical 'motoric' subtypes have been described based on arousal and psychomotor behaviour, as shown in Table 3.1.

It has been demonstrated that the pure hyperactive form of delirium with which we are all very familiar presents in the minority of cases. Lipowski, who formally defined the different subtypes in 1989, was quite clear that despite the fact that

Table 3.1 The three clinical subtypes of delirium that have been described based on arousal and psychomotor behaviour

1	Hyperactive	Hyperaroused	Agitated
2	Hypoactive	Hypoalert	Lethargic
3	Mixed – alternating features of agitation and lethargy		

these patients have varying motoric profiles, they all have the same psychopathological syndrome: delirium. The hypoactivity does not preclude 'intense fantasy life' and terrifying delusions. So the motoric subtype refers to the psychomotor behaviour of the patient and the level of decreased or increased arousal. Consciousness has two components, level of arousal and awareness or understanding of the environment, i.e. cognition. The classic clouding of consciousness in delirium refers to a patient's inability to interact with the environment as well as wakefulness.

There have been attempts to link the pathophysiology and the presentation of delirium. There is little evidence of specific electroencephalogram (EEG) patterns, but a general slowing of EEG waves is common regardless of the delirium subtype (Figure 3.1).

Regarding pathophysiology and one motoric subtype or another, there is speculation about particular neural pathways or lateralization as well as hypotheses about various neurotransmitters. There is not enough known, however, to draw robust conclusions.

Psychomotor behaviour

A delirious patient may display a whole spectrum of motor speed, ranging from hypoactivity to hyperactivity. This is what the motoric subtypes are about.

In **hypoactivity** the patient has a reduced speed in initiating and continuing movements, both spontaneous and

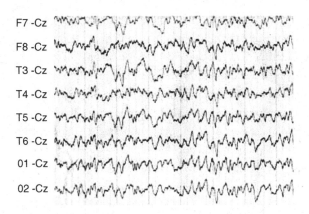

Figure 3.1 Standard electroencephalographic tracing showing a diffusely slow record obtained from a confused patient. There is also increased amplitude of the slow-wave activity on the left side (more in the frontal (F7) and temporal (T3) regions), suggesting the possibility of a problem and necessitating an imaging procedure. Adapted with permission from Boutros NN and Coburn K. Electroencephalography in neuropsychiatry. *Psychiatric Times* 2006; 23. www. psychiatrictimes.com.

when completing a command. Also there is a reduction in the number of spontaneous movements – a still patient.

Conversely, the **hyperactive** patient has an increased number of spontaneous movements as well as moving more quickly, as anyone caught by a flailing arm will testify. The cardinal features of this hyperactive psychomotor behaviour are that it is largely purposeless, uncontrollable and inefficient.

The motoric variant depends on the predominant psychomotor activity and the patient with a **mixed** delirium will fluctuate between hyperactivity and hypoactivity.

Mrs A was a 64-year-old woman admitted to the medical ward with an acute exacerbation of chronic obstructive pulmonary disease. She lived alone following the death of her husband 3 years earlier. Her normal medication was low-dose prednisolone, bronchodilators in inhalers, antihypertensives and ranitidine which were all continued. She was hypoxic on admission and treated with oxygen therapy. All her blood tests were normal apart from a raised C-reactive protein. On the chest radiograph, there was a right basilar shadow and she was started on ciprofloxacin for a presumed infection.

After 3 days, Mrs A became progressively depressed, inhibited and non-compliant with therapy and routine interventions. She was assessed and referred to a psychiatrist for 'depression impairing co-operation and compliance'. On mental status examination she appeared extremely inhibited and apathetic with decreased reaction to stimuli. She had a reduced ability to maintain attention, short-term memory impairment and mild perception disturbances. There was a history of sleep/wake disturbance from the nursing notes. According to her son, she had no cognitive problems before her admission. A diagnosis of hypoactive delirium was made. This was an acute onset of a disturbance in consciousness, attention, cognition and perception.

This had been precipitated by ciprofloxacin and once it was stopped her mental status improved.

(Adapted from Grassi *et al.* [5].)

Hypoactive delirium is often unrecognized or misdiagnosed as sedation or depression. This is even more of a risk in our critical care patients. Lethargy and flat affect is the face of hypoactive delirium. Remember a patient who appears fatigued or with a low mood may in fact be delirious.

Mrs B was a 66-year-old woman who suffered an in-hospital cardiac arrest while recovering from a failed angioplasty. She had emergency coronary bypass grafting, and suffered cardiogenic shock in the early post-operative phase. She then failed to fully regain consciousness during a 28-day course. Continued roving eye movements were noted, with intermittent semi-purposeful writhing motions for which wrist restraints and lorazepam were prescribed. Her husband described an episode of her looking around wildly, trying to scream and fighting to get loose then the nurses rushing in to 'give her a shot'. At other times she was fully comatose. The husband described 'appropriate' gestures, nods and feeble hand grasps but these were not witnessed by any ICU staff. A diagnosis of severe hypoxic brain injury was made and it was suggested that treatment was withdrawn, at which stage the husband asked for her to be transferred to another specialist hospital.

On admission to this other hospital, she was given flumazenil to assess the possibility of a drug-induced coma. After four doses of 0.2 mg intravenously she became more responsive, opening her mouth and protruding her tongue to command. On capping off her tracheostomy tube after deflating the cuff she was able to tell the team her name and where she lived.

This patient had drug-induced delirium cycling with drug-induced coma (Figure 3.2). *She has since returned home.*

(Adapted from Dunn *et al.* [6].)

Mr K was a 70-year-old man who underwent a carotid endarterectomy under local anaesthetics and minimal sedation. He had a number of risk factors predisposing him to developing delirium, which were associated with his generalized vascular disease.

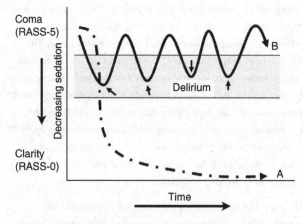

Figure 3.2 This figures represents 'tail-chasing' as a patient starts to wake up into a drug-induced agitated delirious state and is then resedated with benzodiazepine to a drug-induced coma. The arrows represent lorazepam redosing for agitation. The presumed clinical course is shown as line A but what happens most of the time is line B – or the tail-chasing phenomenon. Reprinted with permission of the American Thoracic Society, Copyright American Thoracic Society. Dunn WF *et al.* Iatrogenic delirium and coma: a near miss. *Chest* 2008; 133: 1217–20.

He became slightly confused temporarily during the surgery. In the recovery room, he became acutely agitated, thrashing and pulling at lines while trying to climb out of bed. He was given intravenous haloperidol, more haloperidol, intramuscular olanzapine and a small dose of midazolam to limited effect. He was given a dose of fentanyl but his agitation could only be controlled with small boluses of propofol. Following arrival on the critical care unit he continued to be uncontrollable and a danger to his own safety as well as the staff.

He was given ondansetron and sodium valproate, attempts were made to normalize the environment by removing electrocardiogram monitoring, dimming the lights while calmly reassuring him. The urinary catheter was left in. His QTc had remained within normal limits and he was given more haloperidol with no improvement. It was only when he was sedated with propofol and unresponsive to a verbal stimulus that agitation was controlled. He was eventually intubated and ventilated overnight, remaining sedated with propofol. A brain CT scan was normal. The following morning he was woken up and extubated without issue, having fully recovered and with no memory of his episode of hyperactive delirium.

Mr V was an 80-year-old man who required intubation and ventilation following a complex abdominal surgical intervention. He had a history of gout and hypertension; and had non-insulin-dependent diabetes. He had failed a spontaneous breathing trial on the second post-operative day due to a rising carbon dioxide with worsening acidosis. His delirium assessment (CAM-ICU) in the early afternoon was positive for delirium; he squeezed on all ten letters and had a reduced level of consciousness. That evening he became very restless and pulled out an intravenous line, he was given a bolus of fentanyl, restarted on propofol and given a dose of intravenous haloperidol. He developed a temperature and required increased levels of oxygen. A ventilator-associated pneumonia was diagnosed and he was started on antibiotics. During the night he required another dose of haloperidol for agitation. The following morning the sedation was turned off but he remained difficult to rouse until early evening. He was restless on and off for the next night, requiring even more haloperidol. The following day he was still drowsy but CAM-ICU negative. This patient had suffered classic mixed delirium precipitated by infection and characterized by sleep–wake disturbances.

Prevalence of motoric subtypes

The problem with the main studies in the literature evaluating the subtypes of delirium is the definition. There are several scales or checklists to establish the motoric variant, some better than others. The consistent finding though is that the hypoactive subtype is the most common one.

Outside the critical care unit approximately half of the patients present with hypoactive delirium. On adding together the number of patients with mixed variant delirium and the hypoactive variant delirium you can account for around 80% of all cases.

In the critical care studies to date that have reported on the subtypes of delirium the number of patients with hyperactive delirium is even smaller than in the general hospital population. The fact is that the hyperactive patients are the ones we remember as they can be a danger to themselves and to staff. Hyperactive patients draw our attention with symptoms such as non-co-operation, combativeness, fast or loud speech and wandering. But patients with hyperactive delirium have shorter hospital stays and better outcomes than either mixed or hypoactive subtypes.

In palliative care there is a real concern about missing delirium. One study in Scotland [7] covering eight palliative care units found that 30% of inpatients were delirious; the majority (at least three quarters) had the hypoactive variant. In addition, all available predictive studies show that an age greater than 80 years old is a constant predictor of hypoactive delirium.

Motoric subtypes in critical care and the Richmond Agitation-Sedation Scale

The **R**ichmond **A**gitation-**S**edation **S**cale (RASS) is a 10-point sedation score centred at 0 which means alert and calm (Table 3.2).

Positive RASS scores indicate restlessness (+1), agitation (+2 to +3), or combative behaviour (+4). Negative RASS scores represent lethargy (−1), poor response to verbal stimulus (−2 to −3), responsive only to physical stimulus (−4) and unresponsive (−5). Once the patient is screened positive for delirium using the screening tool Confusion Assessment

Table 3.2 Richmond Agitation-Sedation Scale

+4	Combative	Overly combative, violent, danger to staff
+3	Very agitated	Pulls or removes tube(s) or catheter(s), aggressive
+2	Agitated	Frequent non-purposeful movement, fights ventilator
+1	Restless	Anxious, but movements not aggressive or vigorous
0	Alert and calm	
−1	Drowsy	Not fully alert, but has sustained awakening (eye opening/eye contact) to voice for more than 10 seconds, on verbal stimulation
−2	Light sedation	Briefly awakens with eye contact to voice, for less than 10 seconds, on verbal stimulation
−3	Moderate sedation	Movement or eye opening to voice (but no eye contact), on verbal stimulation
−4	Deep sedation	No response to voice, but movement or eye opening to physical stimulation
−5	Non-arousable	No response to voice or physical stimulation

Adapted with permission from Sessler CN *et al*. The Richmond Agitation-Sedation Scale: validity and reliability in adult intensive care unit patients. *Journal of Respiratory and Critical Care Medicine* 2002; 116: 1338–44.

Method for the ICU (CAM-ICU), the motoric subtype can be largely classified using the RASS. Hyperactive delirium is considered present when the RASS is persistently positive. Hypoactive delirium is defined with a persistently neutral or negative RASS. The mixed type is defined as a delirium episode with both positive and negative RASS values.

In a large series using the above-described method, delirium was detected in 72% of patients older than 64 years old and 57% of younger patients. The proportion of each subtype is shown in Figure 3.3. Older age has been strongly and independently associated with hypoactive delirium [8].

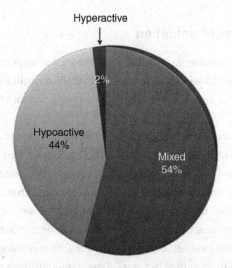

Figure 3.3 Proportion of motoric subtypes amongst delirious patients. Adapted from Peterson JF *et al*. Delirium and its motoric subtypes: a study of 614 critically ill patients. *Journal of the American Geriatrics Society* 2006; 54: 479–84.

In another study, including patients with trauma and in intensive care, in the 59% who were delirious, the proportion of delirium motor subtypes was slightly different with hyperactive in 15%, hypoactive in 46% and mixed in 39%. While the hyperactive variant draws attention by having a higher rate of recorded adverse events (such as self-extubation), there were more patients with hypoactive delirium. These will have issues associated with immobility that increases the length of time on the ventilator, the incidence of infections and pressure sores.

Dilemma of definition

While studies into the prevalence of motoric subtypes are often consistent in their findings, there is concern regarding the variation of tools used to classify the motoric variant of delirium.

There are three often-cited delirium psychomotor checklists used outside critical care (based on Lipowski's description, the Liptzin and Levkoff scheme and the O'Keefe and Lavan scheme); but other studies use pure motor items from a standardized delirium rating scale or a visual analogue scale. So while clinical researchers are working on subgroups and the relationship between duration, outcomes, aetiology and pathophysiology, they lack a validated rating instrument. Those that exist tend to have no clear cut-off values for symptoms' presence or severity and include non-motor symptoms that are of uncertain value, such as irritability and screaming. It is telling that when the three delirium psychomotor checklists and the Delirium Rating Scale-Revised-98 were all applied to a number of patients with delirium there was only agreement 34% of the time!

A scale based on the Delirium Motoric Checklist was developed by Meagher in an attempt to solve this (Table 3.3). It focuses on motor disturbances with four hyperactive items and seven hypoactive items and was validated against subjects without delirium in a study involving patients from a palliative care centre. Although rarely utilized, it is useful to consider it as it focuses on the motor differences between the subtypes.

Aetiology and motoric subtypes

A number of studies have tried to link the cause of delirium to whether it is hyperactive, hypoactive or mixed. Most authors have found no relationship between the motoric type of the delirious patient and the cause. However, some authors suggest that delirium due to alcohol or drug withdrawal is more likely to be hyperactive, while delirium due to metabolic causes is more likely to be hypoactive. These are similar to the observations of a bedside clinician who would predict that the hyperactive type does correlate with alcohol or drug withdrawal, or drug intoxication; and the hypoactive form is linked to hypoxia, metabolic disturbances or when an anticholinergic mechanism is thought to be the trigger. Another small problem is that of the identification of a proper

Table 3.3 Delirium Motoric Checklist as suggested by Meagher. A minimum of two symptoms is needed to meet a subtype criterion

---

Hyperactive subtype If definite evidence in the previous 24 hours of (and this should be a deviation from pre-delirious baseline) at least two of:

Increased quantity of motor activity

Loss of control of activity

Restlessness

Wandering

Hypoactive subtype If definite evidence in the previous 24 hours of (and this should be a deviation from pre-delirious baseline) at least two of (where at least one of either decreased amount of activity or speed of actions is present):

Decreased amount of activity

Decreased speed of actions

Reduced awareness of surroundings

Decreased amount of speech

Decreased speed of speech

Listlessness

Reduced alertness, withdrawal

Mixed motor subtype

If evidence of both hyperactive and hypoactive subtype in the previous 24 hours

No motor subtype

If evidence of neither hyperactive nor hypoactive subtype in the previous 24 hours

---

Adapted with permission from Meagher D *et al*. A new data-based motor subtype schema for delirium. *Journal of Neuropsychiatry and Clinical Neurosciences* 2008; 20: 185–93.

link between cause and motoric type because it is often not possible to identify with certitude a single cause.

Of note, there has been no clear link shown between infection, a common precipitant of delirium, and a particular motoric subtype.

Psychotic symptoms and motoric subtypes

Traditionally it is thought that patients with hypoactive delirium are less likely to suffer hallucinations and delusions. This is not entirely true and these symptoms are more frequent than initially described in patients who are hypoactive.

Perceptual disturbances and delusions are significantly associated with delirium-associated patient distress and therefore important to recognize (and treat) in all delirious patients.

Outcomes and motoric subtypes

The hyperactive type of delirium has the best prognosis, including the highest prospect of full recovery. Outside critical care, the mixed subtype has the worst treatment response and

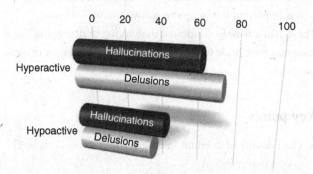

Figure 3.4 **Proportion of hallucinations and delusions according to motoric subtypes.**

hence the worst prognosis. Patients with hypoactive delirium do appear to have longer stays in hospital and may be at risk of increased short-term mortality although that is yet to be proven.

General predictors of outcome, not directly related to motoric type, are older age, longer duration of the episode, pre-existing cognitive impairment and severe physical illness.

Subsyndromal delirium

Lipowski first wrote about subsyndromal delirium, a condition where a patient has some symptoms of delirium but does not meet the full criteria for the diagnosis of delirium. It occurs in patients with similar risks to those who develop delirium and is associated with clinical outcomes that are intermediate between normal and delirious patients. The mortality and ICU length of stay are intermediate for the subsyndromal group, between the clinically delirious and the no delirium patients.

It is important not to ignore subsyndromal delirium. These patients need continued monitoring to determine the direction their brain function is heading – normality or clinical delirium?

Key points

- The majority of delirium in critically ill patients is 'quiet' hypoactive or mixed.
- Hypoactive delirium can be mistaken for sedation or depression.

- Hypoactive delirium is more common in the elderly.
- Hyperactive delirium is associated with better outcomes.

FURTHER READING

Breitbart W and Alici Y. Agitation and delirium at the end of life: "we couldn't manage him". *Journal of the American Medical Association* 2008; 300: 2898-910.

Dunn WF *et al*. Iatrogenic delirium and coma: a near miss. *Chest* 2008; 133: 1217-20.

Meagher D. Motor subtypes of delirium: past, present and future. *International Review of Psychiatry* 2009; 21: 59-73.

Stagno D *et al*. The delirium subtypes: a review of prevalence, phenomenology, pathophysiology and treatment response. *Palliative and Supportive Care* 2004; 2: 171-9.

Chapter 4

Delirium in critical care: how does it happen?

Questions waiting for answers

This chapter is a summary of what is known or suspected about the pathophysiology of delirium. What actually goes on in the brain? How does this explain the symptoms of delirium? And, importantly, how does the mechanism of delirium account for the adverse outcomes?

All good questions. Unfortunately we still do not have the answers.

The pathophysiology of delirium continues to be poorly understood. Reading about delirium pathophysiology leaves the reader frustrated, not knowing what is real, or important or the result of another process.

A number of theories have emerged, including cell membrane stability; oxygen supply and utilization; imbalance of one, two or many neurotransmitters; false transmitters; stress hormones; cytokines; inflammation; blood supply; functional connection disruption; thalamic dysfunction and quite a few more...

Some or all might be true, or linked to the truth. Given the nature of delirium it is likely that several mechanisms contribute to its development in patients.

Start at the end, final common pathway?

Delirium is thought to represent a generalized dysfunction of higher cerebral cortical processes. Not all areas of the brain, however, are equally impaired. Because of its multifactorial nature, it is thought that delirium from different causes may have different mechanisms and/or involve different parts of the brain. The core symptoms may result from the involvement of a final common neural pathway.

A number of core symptoms are commonly found and include sleep–wake cycle disturbances, disorientation and attention deficits. The areas of the brain that aid thinking processes, language and different components of perception and reasoning are implicated in delirium: the frontal, temporal, parietal cortices and their subcortical connections. Less commonly occurring symptoms may mean that some areas of the brain are only affected in certain circumstances. The final common pathway theory suggests that while the appearance of some symptoms may depend on the cause(s), a final common neural disruption is likely to be responsible for core symptoms.

In the frame, oxidative stress

The leading hypotheses for the pathogenesis of delirium include the roles of neurotransmission, inflammation and chronic stress – all of which may result from, or cause, decreased oxidative metabolism. A neuronal ageing hypothesis is added to these, with molecular genetics being able to shed light on underlying metabolic and molecular mechanisms.

It may be that the known causative factors for delirium act by causing changes to neuronal membrane function. These abnormalities of function and polarization result in loss of membrane stability that spreads to neighbouring neurones. This has been called a 'spreading depression'. Neuroimaging in delirium research certainly supports this generalized, cascading effect in the brain, rather than a localized disruption.

Direct brain insults

Processes that cause energy deprivation in areas of the brain are expected to compromise function. These include hypoxia, metabolic derangements, such as those resulting from renal failure or liver impairment, strokes, infection, tumours and drugs.

Inadequate oxidative metabolism may be the cause of the inability to maintain ionic gradients, lead to abnormal neurotransmitter synthesis or disrupt the metabolism of neurotoxic by-products. We know that systemic processes such as hypoxia and hypoglycaemia lead to inattention and loss of cognition, but whether some brain areas are essential for attention and are particularly vulnerable to these effects is uncertain. Localized energy deprivation caused by vascular events in regions essential for attention may also cause delirium.

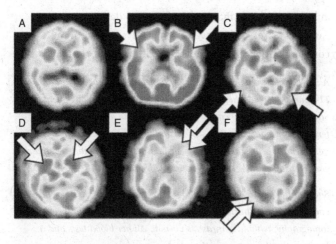

Figure 4.1 Example of single photon emission computed tomography (SPECT) perfusion changes in study patients with delirium. A, normal; B, bilateral frontal hypoperfusion; C, bilateral parietal hypoperfusion; D, hyperperfusion of subcortical structures (seen normally with ageing); E, left frontal hypoperfusion; F, right parietal hypoperfusion. Adapted with permission from Fong TG *et al*. Cerebral perfusion changes in older delirious patients using 99mTc HMPAO SPECT. *Journals of Gerontology. Series A, Biological Sciences and Medical Sciences* 2006; 61: 1294–9.

What can neuroimaging studies tell us?

Research using neuroimaging is limited by the absence of baseline imaging obtained before symptoms, to allow for comparison with long-term outcomes. Brain imaging such as computed tomography scanning (CT scan) can identify anatomical lesions that may be linked to delirium in some cases, e.g. strokes. However, normal CT scans are more common in delirious patients.

A 53-year-old woman is admitted in the emergency room with an 11-hour-long headache. Her sister said she is 'not acting like herself'. Shortly after arrival in casualty she is screaming and combative. Her temperature is measured at 38.8 °C and her heart rate at 157 bpm. Her past medical history includes non-insulin-dependent diabetes, a treated endometrial carcinoma and ongoing depression.

She requires benzodiazepines and haloperidol in order to be calmed enough to allow clinical examination. An emergency cerebral computed tomography, without contrast, is normal. All her blood tests and a lumbar puncture are normal.

A few hours later, she starts suffering hyperactive delirium, thrashing all four limbs and talking incoherently. She requires more drugs to keep her calm.

On the second day she has a magnetic resonance imaging of the brain (Figure 4.2). *This shows small areas of acute infarction in both cerebral hemispheres with numerous foci particularly in the distribution of the left posterior cerebral artery. Stenosis of the carotid arteries, left proximal middle cerebral arteries and left posterior cerebral arteries are visualized.*

She is intubated on day 2 and remains stuporous, restless and confused until day 8. Suddenly, on day 11, she is not delirious anymore and improves to be later discharged.

(Reprinted from the *Journal of Emergency Medicine*, Vol. 24, Vatsavayi V and Malhotra KS, Agitated delirium with posterior cerebral artery infarction, pp. 263–6, Copyright 2003, with permission from Elsevier.)

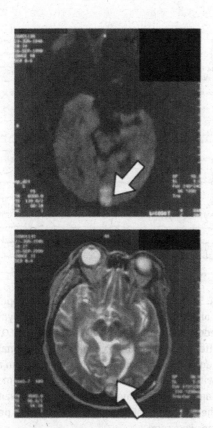

Figure 4.2 Cerebral computed tomography (top) and magnetic resonance imaging (bottom) obtained in the patient described in this case report. Arrows indicate areas of ischaemic changes. Reprinted from the *Journal of Emergency Medicine*, Vol. 24, Vatsavayi V, Malhotra KS., Agitated delirium with posterior cerebral artery infarction, pp. 263–6, Copyright 2003, with permission from Elsevier.

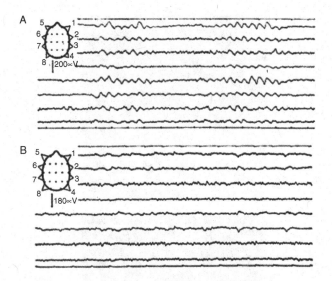

Figure 4.3 A. Severe delirium associated with bronchopneumonia in a woman of 60 years of age. EEG shows bilaterally synchronous frontally predominant 2 Hz runs of delta activity. The EEG returned to normal after recovery. B. Senile dementia in a woman of 80 years of age. EEG shows dominant posterior rhythm at 7–8 Hz associated with irregular theta components, and eye movement artefacts in anteriorly recording channels. Despite advanced dementia, the EEG abnormality is slight. Adapted with permission from www.answers.com.

Hyperactive delirium is common with posterior artery infarction characterized by forced crying out and unintelligible speech. Delirium may be the only sign.

Studies using magnetic resonance imaging (MRI) with diffusion tensor imaging (DTI) on critically ill patients have shown an association between delirium duration and white matter disruption. White matter consists mostly of myelinated axons. White matter integrity is required to control consciousness and attention. Unsurprisingly the white matter disruption is associated with worse cognitive scores up to 12 months later. MRI data show that longer duration of delirium is associated with smaller brain volumes up to 3 months after discharge, and that smaller brain volumes are associated with long-term cognitive impairment at 12 months.

Electroencephalography (EEG)

The electroencephalogram (EEG) records the electrical activity of the brain. A bilateral diffuse abnormality in the electrical background activity is seen in delirium.

The most common findings are a slowing of peak and average frequencies, decreased alpha activity and increased theta and delta waves. Patients with delirium superimposed on dementia show the most abnormal recordings.

EEG parameters are useful in diagnosing delirium in a general population but it is a relatively extensive and time-consuming (and in any case not always available) method for use in daily clinical practice. Conversely when EEG recordings were collected in critically ill patients as part of a sleep study, the predominance of atypical recordings was such that there was a dissociation between the EEG findings and whether a patient was observed to be awake or asleep. This decreases the usefulness of EEG in this setting.

Cerebral blood flow is thought to correlate with metabolic indicators of brain activity such as glucose utilization. Delirium is mostly associated with a decrease in blood flow which usually recovers after the symptoms resolve. One study demonstrated around 40% globally decreased flow during delirium, with greater flow reduction in subcortical structures and occipital cortex compared to other regions.

A story of neuromediators

An imbalance of neurotransmitters is observed in delirium, and may well be the cause of it, whether as a result of neuroinflammation, a lack of oxygen or a drug effect. Extensive evidence supports the role of a central cholinergic deficiency. Deterioration in attention or consciousness also can be linked to an excess of dopamine, but as both acetylcholine and dopamine play a crucial interlinking role, we don't really know which is more important.

Dopamine, norepinephrine and serotonin (5-hydroxytryptamine) have roles in arousal and the sleep–wake cycle, mediating responses to stimuli that are modulated by the cholinergic pathway. Several metabolic pathways lead to significant increases of dopamine under impaired oxidative conditions.

Anatomically the dopaminergic and cholinergic pathways overlap significantly. The prefrontal cortex has six layers of distinct neurotransmitter receptors with various interactions. For example, dopamine inhibits acetylcholine synthesis within layer five by binding onto D2 receptors. Various dopamine receptors impact acetylcholine levels differently.

Serotonin is both directly and indirectly related to cholinergic deficiency. It also stimulates dopaminergic activity. Excess norepinephrine has been associated with hyperactive delirium. Norepinephrine controls some dopaminergic neurones as well as interfacing with cholinergic pathways.

GABA (γ-aminobutyric acid) activity typically depresses neuronal excitability. An interesting theory regarding drug-induced delirium is that it is caused by a temporary dysfunction of the thalamic filtering regulated by GABA receptors. This makes sense when one knows that the thalamus plays a key role in processing and integrating sensory information relevant to emotional and cognitive functions.

Benzodiazepines and propofol are alike in that they are GABA-ergic in action and acutely impair cognitive function. Benzodiazepines in particular are strongly implicated in causing delirium.

Of note, GABA activity is implicated in hepatic encephalopathy and flumazenil, a benzodiazepine antagonist, has been shown to reverse coma and improve hypoactive delirium in cirrhotic patients (although with no effect on recovery or survival).

Serum anticholinergic activity (SAA)

A serum biomarker for delirium would be extremely useful as an objective parameter in diagnosing delirium. If it is assumed that there is an imbalance in dopaminergic and cholinergic

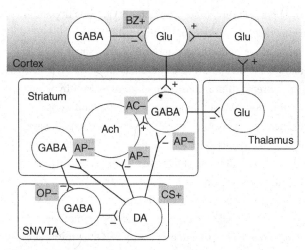

Figure 4.4 Schematic diagram illustrating the pathways and sites of action of psychotogenic and antipsychotic agents. The psychotic symptoms of drug-induced delirium would originate from a transitory thalamic dysfunction leading to sensory overload and hyperarousal. Certain psychoactive medications frequently prescribed to hospitalized patients can contribute to the generation/exacerbation (anticholinergics – AC, benzodiazepines – BZ, corticosteroids – CS, opioids – OP) or improvement (antipsychotics – AP) of psychotic symptoms. SN/VTA, substantia nigra–ventral tegmental area; Glu, glutamate; Ach, acetylcholine; DA, dopamine. Adapted with permission from Gaudreau JD and Gagnon P. Psychotogenic drugs and delirium pathogenesis: the central role of the thalamus. *Medical Hypotheses* 2005; 64(3): 471–5.

neurotransmitter systems and peripheral serum anticholinergic activity (SAA) levels adequately reflect central anticholinergic change, then the detection of high anticholinergic activity in the serum should be associated with delirious symptoms. The normal healthy person does not have detectable SAA activity and some have suggested that measurement of SAA levels is a reliable indicator of delirium. However, it is likely that treatment with anticholinergic drugs or other medication that has anticholinergic activity can influence SAA levels. So far, its measurement in delirious patients has not demonstrated any difference from controls. SAA levels are not a reliable indicator of delirium and dementia in a frail elderly population.

The vulnerable brain

Age and pre-existing cognitive impairment are two well-known risk factors for delirium. A decrease in the volume of acetylcholine-producing cells and a decrease in cerebral oxidative metabolism are observed with age. Both factors lead to a normal decline in acetylcholine synthesis, which may explain why increasing age is an independent predictor of delirium. These normal processes are aggravated by even mild hypoxia, as this further inhibits acetylcholine synthesis and release. Animal studies in an early dementia mouse model have demonstrated that brain cholinergic depletion predisposes to an acute cognitive deficit following a systemic inflammatory insult.

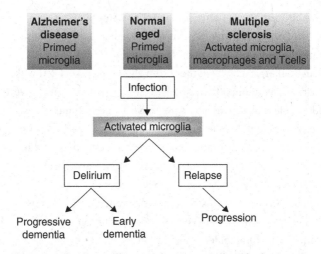

Figure 4.5 The 'normal' ageing brain, as well as the brains of multiple sclerosis (MS) and Alzheimer's disease patients, contains primed microglia. In the case of MS, in addition to overtly activated macrophages and T cells in the plaques, there are many activated microglia in white matter tracts containing degenerating axons. All of these microglia might be further activated by systemic insults to produce neurotoxic compounds, compromising neurones and causing reversible cognitive and/or neurological deficits. This is likely to manifest as a relapse in MS patients and as delirium in normal aged or demented patients. However, the acute exacerbation of inflammation in the central nervous system might also cause permanent damage, facilitating progression of MS-associated neurological deficits and accelerating cognitive decline in the aged or demented patient. Adapted by permission from Macmillan Publishers Ltd. Perry VH *et al*. The impact of systemic infection on the progression of neurodegenerative disease. *Nature Reviews Neuroscience* 2003; 4: 103–12.

Reduction in the activity of cholinergic neurones is a feature of Alzheimer's disease, a disease that carries an increased risk of delirium. In Alzheimer's, metabolic changes (hypoactivation) alongside plaque formation and grey matter atrophy are observed in regions critical to maintaining a normal and clear sensorium. Dementia is also associated with decreased cerebral oxidative metabolism, cholinergic deficiency and inflammation.

With increasing age there is also a broad decline in cardiovascular and respiratory reserves apart from in chronic illnesses seen in the elderly. Over recent years, small-vessel cerebrovascular disease has become increasingly recognized as an important contributor to cognitive and functional decline in elderly people. This may lead to a reduced capacity for compensatory changes with mild hypotension or hypoxia. There is evidence that chronic hypoperfusion induces chronic oxidative damage.

Grey matter atrophy in the elderly brain results in less robust functional connections between areas of the brain. The neuronal circuit involved in general attention is activated and maintained via the ascending reticular activating system arising from the brainstem. Connections are potentially weakened in the critically ill patient by the stress of illness, drugs and other challenges. Minor fluctuations in the ascending reticular activating system may be sufficient to cause disruption and lead to the symptoms of delirium. Prolonged uncoupling of the connections may result in neurodegenerative processes such as excitotoxicity and apoptosis, leaving a patient with long-term cognitive impairment.

Table 4.1 Study demonstrating the benefits of early mobilization. Intervention was sedation breaks with active mobilization from passive limb exercises to active exercises through to sitting as tolerated. Control had only sedation breaks. All in one single centre.

	Intervention n = 49	Control n = 55	p value
Return to independent functional status at hospital discharge	59%	35%	0.02
ICU delirium (days)	2.0 (0.0–6.0)	4.0 (2.0–7.0)	0.03
Time in ICU with delirium	33%	57%	0.02
Hospital delirium (days)	2.0 (0.0–6.0)	4.0 (2.0–8.0)	0.02
Hospital days with delirium	28%	41%	0.01
ICU-acquired paresis at hospital discharge	31%	49%	0.09
Duration of mechanical ventilation (days)	3.4 (2.3–7.3)	6.1 (4.0–9.6)	0.02
Length of stay in ICU (days)	5.9 (2.4–5.5)	7.9 (6.1–14.1)	0.08
Length of stay in hospital (days)	13.5 (8.0–23.1)	12.9 (8.9–19.8)	0.93
Hospital mortality	18%	25%	0.53

Reprinted from the *Lancet* Vol. 373, Issue 9678. Schweickert WD *et al.* Early physical and occupational therapy in mechanically ventilated critically ill patients: a randomised controlled trial, pp. 1874–82, Copyright 2009, with permission from Elsevier.

Interestingly, animal models have demonstrated that immobilization causes widespread acetylcholine reduction. Immobilization is often quoted as being a predisposing risk factor in delirium. Mobilizing patients early, even just sitting on the edge of the bed, decreases not only length of ICU stay but also duration of delirium.

The septic brain

Sepsis is a complex syndrome characterized by an imbalance between the pro- and anti-inflammatory responses to an infection or physiological insult. There is an unregulated systemic response culminating in multiple organ failure, which has a high mortality rate. Up to 71% of septic patients develop acute cerebral dysfunction – generally referred to as septic encephalopathy – this manifests as delirium.

Peripherally measured levels of C-reactive protein, a marker of acute inflammatory response, are higher in patients with delirium. Interleukin 8 is at its highest in the days leading up to delirium in post-operative patients.

In patients with sepsis, acetylcholine activates pathways that inhibit pro-inflammatory cytokine synthesis and protect against both ischaemic–reperfusion injury and endotoxaemia. Deficits in acetylcholine will therefore trigger a neuroinflammatory response.

The brain plays a vital role in the normal functioning of the immune response. Normal communication between the central nervous system and the periphery is necessary to modulate local inflammatory responses. These mechanisms include the release of hypothalamic–pituitary hormones and activation of the sympathetic nervous system. In addition the cholinergic anti-inflammatory pathway is a neural-based

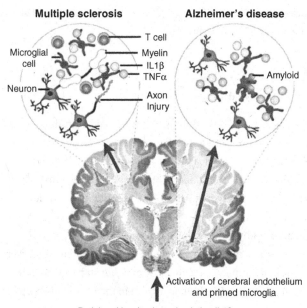

Figure 4.6 In chronic neurodegenerative diseases, such as Alzheimer's disease and multiple sclerosis, peripheral insults that result in elevated peripheral cytokine synthesis can cause the activation of already primed microglia and lead to acute central cytokine synthesis with behavioural consequences. These cytokines, or other secretory products of the activated microglia, might cause axonal or neuronal damage and produce a lasting effect on the neurodegenerative process. IL, interleukin; TNF, tumour necrosis factor. Adapted with permission from Macmillan Publishers Ltd. Perry PH *et al*. The impact of systemic infection on the progression of neurodegenerative disease. *Nature Reviews Neuroscience* 2003; 4: 103–12.

system that leads to the local release of acetylcholine. This neurotransmitter interacts with macrophages to inhibit the release of tumour necrosis factor (TNF) and other pro-inflammatory cytokines. In summary, the normal central nervous system responses act to maximize the defensive capabilities where needed while preventing systemic toxicity.

Clinical and experimental data suggest that there are a number of factors involved, including the local generation of pro-inflammatory cytokines, impaired cerebral microcirculation, the inevitable imbalance of neurotransmitters and the impact on peripheral organ failure. Diffuse endothelial activation induced by sepsis may result in blood–brain barrier breakdown. Injection of lipopolysaccharide (the active fragment of Gram-negative bacteria) and cytokines peripherally or centrally causes cognitive impairments and behavioural disturbances in both animals and humans.

Exposing brains to lipopolysaccharide leads to decrease of regional cerebral blood flow in the cortex and to microglial activation (the microglia include the resident macrophages in the brain and are a major source of inflammatory molecules). Cerebral microcirculatory failure and systemic and local inflammation mutually influence neuronal activity and promote each other during sepsis. This is contrary to early assumptions that the brain was protected by the blood–brain barrier, a lack of lymph system and a lack of histocompatibility complex antigen on the parenchyma cells. The brain is in fact profoundly affected by the peripheral immune system. When the brain is already damaged by an ongoing neurodegenerative disease such as Alzheimer's disease, the disruption is likely to be more severe.

Regarding the impact of delirium on outcomes, including death, it has been suggested that the central nervous system dysfunction may contribute to the pathogenesis of severe sepsis, firstly through the impairment of neural-based pathways for inter-organ and intercellular communication, in particular haemodynamic responses. Also signalling within the brain and between the brain and the periphery maintains normal immune responses. This loss of physiological control and modulation may be a fundamental cause of multiple organ impairment where a decrease in central nervous system anti-inflammatory mechanisms results in an overproduction of inflammatory mediators at local sites. There is evidence that systemic infections and therefore cytokine production may enhance neurodegeneration when neuronal damage is already present, for instance with stroke or multiple sclerosis.

Delirium and cortisol

Glucocorticoids are fundamental to the stress response. Dysfunction of the stress response and heightened inflammatory states are common with ageing and neurodegeneration. A dysfunctional stress response is listed as a major mechanism of delirium, alongside direct brain insults involving energy deprivation, metabolic disturbance or direct trauma to brain tissues. This can be either an abnormally intense response with increased or sustained levels of cortisol and other signalling molecules, or an exaggerated response of the brain to normal stimuli.

In demented patients, basal cortisol levels are significantly different in various groups of patients with differing severities of delirium. Early in stroke, delirium is associated with an increased adrenocortical sensitivity due to an increased stimulation by adrenocorticotrophic hormone, resulting from an impaired negative-feedback mechanism.

Excessive glucocorticoid levels seem to induce a vulnerable state in neurones, with the hippocampus as principal target.

Be warned, steroids may not be good for your patient's brain when you have the delirium mindset!

Delirium and amino acids

Precursors of cerebral neurotransmitters include the amino acids tryptophan, phenylalanine and tyrosine. Changes in the cerebral availability of these particular amino acids affect the production of neurotransmitters.

Both an increase and a decrease in serotonin levels are associated with delirium. The rate of serotonin production is dependent on the availability of the precursor tryptophan. There is competition between tryptophan and the 'other large neutral amino acids' (oLNAA). Tryptophan competes with oLNAA such as tyrosine, phenylalanine and valine for transport across the blood–brain barrier – they all use the same saturable carrier. The ratio of tryptophan to oLNAA ultimately determines the production of serotonin. In patients who develop delirium following cardiac surgery, plasma tryptophan and the tryptophan:oLNAA ratio are decreased. Whether the association occurs secondary to increased serotonin concentrations in the brain or via the downstream production of neurotoxic metabolites is not known.

Phenylalanine is a precursor of dopamine and norepinephrine through a tyrosine connection. Levels of tyrosine and phenylalanine relative to the oLNAA determine the amount of amino acids that reaches the brain. Increase in tyrosine and phenylalanine uptake may be a risk factor for delirium as this will increase dopamine and norepinephrine production. In cardiac surgery, the ratio of phenylalanine to oLNAA is increased in patients who became delirious; low or high levels of tryptophan:oLNAA and tyrosine:oLNAA ratios are significantly associated with transitioning to delirium in ventilated patients.

Liver dysfunction results in decreased metabolism of the precursor amino acids leading to an increase in tryptophan and consequently serotonin. Elevated tryptophan availability and increased cerebral serotonin is in turn associated with hepatic encephalopathy.

Immunology and genetics

Insulin-like growth factor 1 (IGF-1) and somatostatin are neurotrophic peptides integral to the growth and survival of neurones and important in the context of cognition.

A reversible somatostatin reduction is seen in delirious patients. Brain cells release cytokines in response to an insult and some of these will inhibit IGF-1 activity and influence cell survival. The neuroprotective influence of these peptides is shown in several studies including patients post brain injury.

Researchers have been working on the relationship between patient's genes and predisposition to delirium with conflicting results. Apolipoprotein E4 (*ApoE4*) genotype (as opposed to *ApoE2* and *ApoE3* allele) is present in 14% of the population and is identified as a major susceptibility factor for Alzheimer's disease. It is associated with poor neurological outcome after

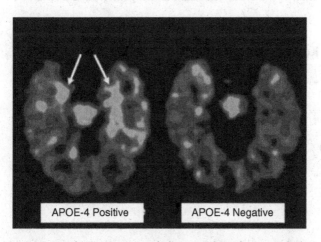

Figure 4.7 PET brain scans reveal plaque and tangle accumulation in patients with the *ApoE4* gene, which increases risk of Alzheimer's. Photo: Courtesy of UCLA, © UCLA. From website Virtual Medical Worlds Monthly: www.hoise.com/vmw/09/repository/PET_brain.jpg.

closed head injury and intracranial haemorrhage. One hypothesis is that the ApoE4 isoform is less effective at suppressing central nervous system inflammation than the ApoE2 or ApoE3 isoforms.

Other genes that regulate the metabolism of certain neurotransmitters have been implicated in the development of delirium. Catechol-*O*-methyltransferase (COMT) is an essential enzyme for the synthesis and breakdown of dopamine in the prefrontal cortex and exists in different genetic variants. Individual differences in the metabolism of dopamine may be related to differential outcomes for acute brain dysfunction, cell death and cognitive impairment.

Key points

- Neurotransmitter imbalance is present in delirium – a relative cholinergic-deficient state with excess dopamine.
- Neurotransmitter imbalance has many possible causes, direct or indirect, and results in oxidative stress.
- Elderly brains are more vulnerable.
- There are no clinically useful blood tests or neuroimaging investigations currently available to diagnose delirium.

FURTHER READING

Quarterly newsletter of the European Delirium Association highlights the latest important research in delirium. www.europeandeliriumassociation.com/.

Maldonado JR. Pathoetiological model of delirium: a comprehensive understanding of the neurobiology of delirium and an evidence-based approach to prevention and treatment. *Critical Care Clinics* 2008; 24(4): 789–856.

Trzepacz P. The neuropathogenesis of delirium. A need to focus our research. *Psychosomatics* 1994; 35(4): 374–9.

Chapter 5

Delirium: what causes it? Risk factors

Introduction

Delirium is serious. A good clinician is keen to reduce the number of patients who develop this syndrome. But what causes delirium? Are some patients more susceptible than others? Should we routinely screen for delirium? If yes, which group of patients?

Good questions but we don't have all the answers... just a few which we will explore in this chapter.

Considering that the pathophysiology is still unclear, it is not surprising that studies to establish what puts a patient more at risk of developing delirium come up with a number of different answers. If we understood the mechanisms, then we would be able to explore with greater accuracy the predisposing and precipitating factors. Risk factors cover a wide range of disparate patient characteristics and illnesses, often related to the various mechanistic hypotheses that include inflammation, lack of oxygen supply, neurotransmitter imbalance caused by drugs, ageing process, or all the above... No fewer than 61 risk factors were identified out of 27 prospective studies including 1365 patients with delirium.

We know that critically ill patients are particularly at risk of delirium and we need to screen all critically ill patients regularly, at least daily. Risk factors can be controlled (to some extent) and delirium can be managed (sometimes) but only if we know it is present.

Delirium studies and statistics

Types of studies

Three main types of clinical studies are done to identify risk factors in developing delirium.

The first ones screen a series of patients prospectively or retrospectively, collecting data on the many variables that have previously been identified as risk factors and others that the clinicians performing the study believe may be important. The data then undergo statistical crunching to confirm which risk factors are significant. A predictive rule or model can then be generated and these allow clinicians to identify which patients are most at risk.

The second group of studies concentrate on a specific factor (such as use of morphine or the level of education). This factor might have been identified in studies such as described above. This factor is then tested as to whether it is significant in the development of delirium. This design was used to generate PRE-DELIRIC, a delirium prediction model for intensive care patients.

The third group is similar to the second, but specific risk factors are studied in a very specific hospital population (e.g.

patients undergoing abdominal surgery or having fractured neck of femur, or both).

Some of these second and third types of studies have been interested in the intensive care patient population but many more have studied other 'at risk' patients, such as the elderly, patients with advanced cancer, or post-operative patients.

Basic statistics

Delirium studies initially look for bi-variable relationships, i.e. each factor is tested for individual significance in patients with and without delirium. A number are then identified as significantly different when delirium is present, for instance a metabolic derangement, history of hypertension or cardiac failure in the 'with delirium' group. These then need to be adjusted for confounding factors. Confounding factors will make a risk factor appear more or less significant than it is. We intuitively know this. Often clinicians say, 'more patients with delirium die because they are sicker; therefore delirium is a marker of illness rather than a predictor of mortality'. Patients with delirium are often sicker so the second test effectively compares patients of the same risk and then sees, with that adjustment, whether the mortality is still significantly higher. And most studies have shown that delirium is an independent predictor of mortality. Similarly with age: older patients may get more delirium so on simple significance testing increasing age is a risk factor. However, because we know impaired cognitive function is a risk factor and elderly patients are more likely to have impaired cognitive function we need to control for cognitive function before we can conclude age is a risk factor.

Controlling for different factors and then testing for each variable in turn makes multivariable analyses complex endeavours even in the world of statistics. Multivariable models refer to statistical techniques dealing with several variables. They adjust for confounding factors and can evaluate the effect of those factors that are significant after confounders are adjusted for. Multivariable analyses are best regarded as a powerful but complex and demanding type of analysis, appropriate to the final stages of a study, rather than as a magical black box to provide a short cut to a result.

The number of patients recruited in any clinical study will vary considerably, with sometimes fewer than 20 subjects enrolled or detected; these studies are likely to be underpowered. As clinicians, however, we will usually consider it likely that even the smallest sample size study includes one or more factors that probably contribute to the development of delirium – but does it mean that it is The Answer? We record and read case reports, and swap stories, but taking firm conclusions from these is considered unscientific, albeit pragmatic.

Studies that do not adjust for confounding factors in delirium will claim that some factors are significant when in fact they are just surrogate markers. Conversely, factors that fail to reach significance in a multivariable analysis still may provide us with valuable information needed to recognize the high-risk patient.

Risk factors are cumulative, and the clinical mind needs to be attentive and wonder if a factor has been excluded because of falling short of probability law or because of the greater effect of another related one. Factors cannot be considered in isolation, and a two-dimensional table is probably not the best way to interpret results as the factors are usually interlinked. Risk model studies help to focus on clinically relevant risk factors that contribute the most to whether a patient will become delirious. Their aim is to identify the level of a patient's risk for developing delirium from either the baseline characteristics and/or a clinical measurement(s). This is similar to risk assessment for thrombosis following which a patient is put into a low-, medium- or high-risk category and prophylaxis decided accordingly.

Predisposing risk factors

Predisposing risk factors refer to those elements that set a patient up to develop delirium, they describe the vulnerable patient. They exist before the patient becomes delirious and the important ones are difficult if not impossible to modify (such as history of delirium, chronic renal failure or having a fracture).

Cognitive impairment and older age are both consistent predisposing factors in non-ICU studies. Both are non-modifiable. The probability of transitioning to delirium in ICU increases dramatically for each year of life after 65 years. Ageing cannot be prevented but cognitive impairment can... perhaps just by reading this book. Some ICU studies have dismissed older age as significant in critically ill patients, but this may just be that the combination of stronger factors pushed age down the probability list.

Dehydration is a known predisposing factor that is modifiable, and aggressive fluid resuscitation may protect patients from delirium.

Non-pharmacological management therapies for delirium are directed at decreasing the impact of predisposing risk

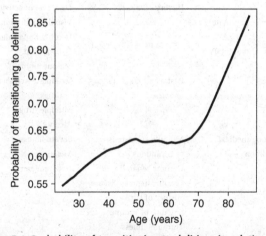

Figure 5.1 Probability of transitioning to delirium in relation to age. Adapted with permission from Pandharipande *et al*. Lorazepam is an independent risk factor for transitioning to delirium in intensive care unit patients. *Anesthesiology* 2006; 104(4): 21–6.

factors, for example making sure a patient has visual aids. Indeed mobilizing ICU patients early has been shown to decrease the number of days they suffer delirium.

Table 5.1 Predisposing risk factors for delirium

	Non-modifiable	Modifiable
Demographic	Age of 65 years or older	
	Male sex	
Cognitive status	Dementia	Depression
	Cognitive impairment	
	History of delirium	
Functional status	Functional dependence	Immobility
	History of falls	Low level of activity
Sensory impairment		Visual impairment
		Hearing impairment
Decreased oral intake		Dehydration
		Malnutrition
Drugs	Past alcohol/substance abuse	Multiple psychoactive drugs
		Multiple drugs
		Alcohol
Coexisting medical condition	Multiple coexisting conditions	Severe illness
	Chronic renal disease	Metabolic derangement
	Chronic hepatic disease	
	History of stroke	
	Fracture or trauma	
	Terminal illness	
	Infection with HIV	

Adapted with permission from Inouye SK *et al.* Delirium in older persons. *New England Journal of Medicine* 2006; 354: 1157–65. Copyright © Massachusetts Medical Society. All rights reserved.

Cognitive decline

The only risk factor consistently identified in or outside ICU is pre-existing cognitive impairment. Cognitive decline is usually diagnosed by using a surrogate assessment of cognitive function from someone (a proxy) who is familiar with the patient. Two tools are commonly used: one looks for cognitive decline over the previous 6 months (a version of the Blessed Dementia Rating Scale); and one looks for cognitive decline over a number of years (the Informant Questionnaire on Cognitive Decline in the Elderly).

When taking a history of a critically ill patient we do not usually ask about degrees of cognitive decline or how the patient has managed day-to-day activities before admission as compared with, say, a year previously. Rather we assume a family member or friend will volunteer any such information regarding pre-existing dementia. Sometimes a patient is mistakenly labelled as having dementia and this has not been questioned. Perhaps it is time to change.

A woman recently admitted to ICU was handed over as having a diagnosis of dementia and acute renal failure. She had been quietly restless and generally uncommunicative. On being assessed using the CAM-ICU, she was able to obey a direct command to squeeze the nurse's hand but on being asked to squeeze only on the letter A in a 10-letter sequence simply tapped the assessor's hand for the first five letters and repeated the letters out loud. The only question she answered in the negative was when asked if a hammer was used to hit a nail. So she screened positive for delirium. Her elderly husband arrived and he told the team that she was usually mobile, looked after herself although was

a little forgetful. He had been unable to get to the hospital before then.
All too often the label of dementia is wrongly applied; given the right
history this patient was clearly delirious from the outset. Her delirium
cleared after a cycle of haemofiltration and a nephrostomy insertion.
Whether a patient has long-term cognitive impairment – or in this case
not – is important to know.

Education

Lack of education can include a greater susceptibility not only
to dementia but to delirium. Among the markers of cognitive
reserve, educational attainment is probably the most analysed.
Some investigators claim that education is the most important
risk factor in dementia.

Cognitive reserve refers to the ability of the brain to function
in the event of damage. It could do so by passive and active
processes. Passive processes refer to the idea of a hypothetical
critical threshold of damage before that injury is seen
clinically. The threshold is greater in some patients than
others. Active processes are explained as the brain actively
attempting to compensate for damage by using alternative
networks or established connections more efficiently.
Education may confer an ability to use the brain more flexibly
providing a greater reserve in the event of damage, acute or
chronic.

In delirium, some studies dismiss education as a risk factor
(although those studies were not designed to demonstrate the
impact of education) – but in elderly patients admitted to an

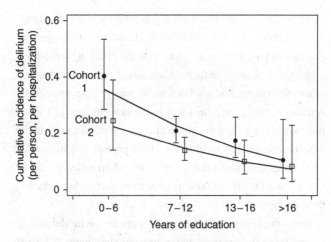

Figure 5.2 Probability of transitioning to delirium in relation to education. Cohort 1 included 491 patients and cohort 2 461 patients. Adapted with permission from Jones RN *et al*. Does educational attainment contribute to risk for delirium? A potential role for cognitive reserve. *Journals of Gerontology. Series A, Biological Sciences and Medical Sciences* 2006; 61: 1307–11.

acute care hospital, the excess risk associated with a 6-year difference in education was equivalent to the presence of dementia.

Risk model in hospitalized patients

In 1993 Sharon Inouye and colleagues looked at elderly medical patients and the relationship between admission characteristics and delirium. They identified 13 variables to test in a multivariate analysis (assessing the contribution of each variable to the risk of getting delirium while controlling for the others). Four variables were identified as independent risk factors (see Table 5.2). From this, they built up a model to identify risk of developing delirium based on a patient's admission characteristics. Each factor was given a score of 1. A patient scoring no points was in the low-risk group, 1 to 2 points in an intermediate group and the remainder were in the high-risk group. The incidence of delirium was 42% in patients with a high risk, and subsequently 26% when tested in an independent cohort of patients. Far from perfect but better than nothing.

The same researchers developed a predictive model for factors following hospitalization, initially identifying 25 factors narrowed down to five final independent variables predicting pre-existing delirium (see Table 5.3).

Table 5.2 Risk model based on patient hospital admission characteristics – elderly medical patients

Risk factor	Adjusted relative risk (95% confidence interval)
Vision impairment	3.51 (1.15–10.71)
Severe illness (APACHE > 16 or nurse rating of severe)	3.49 (1.48–8.23)
Cognitive impairment (Mini Mental State Examination score < 24)	2.82 (1.19–6.65)
Blood urea nitrogen/creatinine ratio > 18	2.02 (0.89–4.60)

Adapted with permission from Inouye SK *et al.* A predictive model for delirium in hospitalized elderly medical patients based on admission characteristics. *Annals of Internal Medicine* 1993; 119: 474–81.

Table 5.3 Risk model based on precipitating factors during hospitalization

Use of physical restraints	1 point
Malnutrition	1 point
> 3 medications added	1 point
Bladder catheter	1 point
Any iatrogenic event	1 point
0 points	Low risk
1-2 points	Intermediate risk
> 2 points	High risk

Reprinted with permission from Inouye SK and Charpentier PA. Precipitating factors for delirium in hospitalized elderly persons: predictive model and interrelationship with baseline vulnerability. *Journal of the American Medical Association* 1996; 275(11): 852–7. Copyright © 1996 American Medical Association. All rights reserved.

Again they used a system of one point per risk factor where three or more precipitating factors puts your patient into a high-risk group – highlighting the cumulative relationship between factors. Because these factors are related to events once in hospital all five of the precipitating factors are potentially modifiable in patients.

PRE-DELIRIC

PRE-DELIRIC was developed and validated in the Netherlands in a study involving five intensive care units and 3056 patients. It uses ten variables (risk factors) collected after 24 hours in intensive care. These are processed into an equation and the result is the percentage chance of an individual patient developing delirium during a critical care stay. The factors that confer the greatest risk are coma from any cause (other than pure drug related), infection and the use of sedatives. It is a valuable resource in critical care units with electronic records. PRE-DELIRIC has some shortcomings, including that it requires a clinician to judge whether a patient is in coma due to sedation, illness or a combination – and the difference can alter the risk considerably. In addition, the formula takes no account of cognitive impairment or alcohol abuse because not enough patients of either group were enrolled while the model was being developed and validated.

PRE-DELIRIC is a useful research tool enabling interventions to be assessed according to patient populations, as an intervention may for example work in patients at high risk but not those at low risk. It may prove useful in clinical practice. PRE-DELIRIC is free to download and use.

Precipitating causes

Delirium always has underlying causes, triggered by events or changes in patient status. An underlying cause is made up of the precipitating factors, such as infection or some medications (interestingly, some medications have a bad reputation even if not always backed up by evidence – see later in this chapter).

Any individual can become delirious given sufficient stimulus – but each individual will react differently and may need more or less activation. Delirium can be triggered in an elderly patient with what would normally be considered a fairly mild insult.

Table 5.4 Precipitating factors for delirium

	Non-modifiable	Modifiable
Drugs		Sedative hypnotics
		Opioids
		Anticholinergic drugs
		Multiple drug therapy
		Alcohol or drug withdrawal
Primary neurological disease	Stroke	
	Intracranial bleeding	
	Meningitis or encephalitis	
Intercurrent illness		Infections
		Iatrogenic complications
		Severe acute illness
		Hypoxia
		Shock
		Fever or hypothermia
		Anaemia
		Dehydration
		Poor nutritional status
		Metabolic derangement
Surgery	Required orthopaedic surgery	
	Required cardiac surgery	Duration of bypass
	Required non-cardiac surgery	
Environment	Required admission to ICU	Use of physical restraints
	Required bladder catheter	
	Required multiple procedure	Pain
		Emotional stress
		Prolonged sleep deprivation

Adapted with permission from Inouye SK. Delirium in older persons. *New England Journal of Medicine* 2006; 354(11): 1157–65. Copyright © Massachusetts Medical Society. All rights reserved.

A 72-year-old diabetic woman who had recovered from pneumonia and was waiting for a ward bed was having difficulty sleeping on the ICU. She was on treatment for hypertension and normally wore glasses but had given them to her daughter to look after while she was in hospital. She was given a dose of temazepam to help her sleep and within 2 hours became acutely confused. By the morning she was back to normal albeit tired! Her delirium had been precipitated by a benzodiazepine.

The degree of vulnerability determined by the patient's baseline characteristics governs how 'strong' a trigger is needed to set off delirium.

It is not always easy to identify a single precipitating cause of delirium, particularly in the elderly population. One study revealed a total of 258 potential causes, or an average of three per patient. Only a few patients had a single precipitating factor identified but several had four factors or more.

It is nearly impossible to rank precipitating factors, but it might not be far from the truth to list infection, acutely altered metabolism, adverse drug effects and cardiovascular events as the most common factors in the elderly. Precipitating factors can be predisposing as well!

Drugs as precipitating factors

Countless drugs have been implicated in causing delirium symptoms... Clinicians believe they already know the drugs that cause delirium, those with an anticholinergic action for a start, but this is not always demonstrated in practice. Scientific (statistical) evidence is lacking.

Benzodiazepines have appeared to be the worst enemy. Lorazepam and midazolam are demonstrated to be risk factors for delirium in medical and surgical ICU patients. Benzodiazepines increase the risk of delirium in hospitalized cancer patients in a dose-related manner. A Cochrane review looking into the use of benzodiazepines in the treatment of agitated delirium concluded that they cannot be recommended in this condition. Every unit dose of lorazepam given in the previous 24 hours is significantly associated with a 20% risk increase in the daily transition to delirium. After 20 mg, there is no further increase... because the risk is then 100%. A study investigating the association of delirium

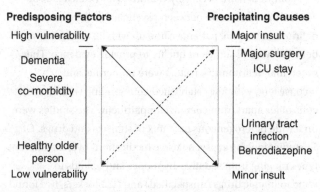

Figure 5.3 Multifactorial model for delirium. The development of delirium involves a complex interrelationship between baseline patient vulnerability (left axis) and precipitating factors or noxious insults occurring during hospitalization. Adapted with permission from Inouye SK. Predisposing and precipitating factors for delirium in hospitalized older patients. *Dementia and Geriatric Cognitive Disorders* 1999; 10: 393–400.

and sedative-induced coma in 99 patients receiving fentanyl and midazolam produced contradictory findings, with delirium being unrelated to midazolam but associated with the inflammatory status. The authors of these studies with apparently conflicting results are to be congratulated for attempting to unpick this complex drugs–brain interaction. Many more pieces of the delirium jigsaw need to come together. We DO know that benzodiazepines are long-acting drugs, and opiates relieve pain.

Other precipitants include commonly prescribed psychoactive medications, such as opioid analgesics, benzodiazepines and corticosteroids.

A comprehensive review by Gaudreau and colleagues in 2005 of the association between psychoactive drugs and delirium in hospital patients came up with 22 studies they believed were of sufficient quality to provide evidence. They noted that delirium risk factors were numerous and inconsistent, with few established confounding variables to control for apart from cognitive impairment. The studies were on a wide heterogeneous case mix of subjects and drugs. Of 11 studies looking at psychoactive medications overall, different types ranging from sedative–hypnotics and opioids to anticholinergic drugs (unspecified) and H2 blockers, five found an increased risk with exposure. Positive results were found for anticonvulsants and antiemetics but this was only on direct statistical testing and confounding factors were not adjusted for. The authors were somewhat critical of the methodological limitations of all the studies and concluded with a list of eight considerations for anyone considering such an enterprise in the future. While none of the three studies into corticosteroids and delirium found an association, a more recent study in patients with acute lung injury has shown steroid use as a risk factor.

Meperidine is a great contender for the worst precipitating drug (thought to be due in part to the neuroexcitatory metabolite normeperidine). Morphine is also a risk factor in cancer patients, sometimes shown be directly linked to the dose. Modifying the dose can sometimes affect the effect. Delirium and visual hallucinations occur at 60 mg but only visual hallucinations at 40 mg.

But while receiving the drug can be the cause, avoiding it can be as bad. Receiving no analgesia or low-dose morphine after hip fracture is associated with an increased risk of delirium. Pain can be associated with a ninefold risk of developing delirium. It is important to note that pain is a risk factor.

In ICU patients two studies have failed to identify a significant association with opioid use and delirium; however, one study on surgical ICU patients showed fentanyl use was a risk factor. The use of benzodiazepines and/or opioids in combination in a relatively large study of 304 patients was significant; specifically, in patients without dementia there was a 142% increase in the rate of delirium. For patients with dementia the positive association was reduced and not significant – confused yet?

Drugs with anticholinergic properties are implicated in causing delirium. Prochlorperazine (Stemetil), theophylline, digoxin, furosemide and isosorbide dinitrate are all possible culprits. In fact 14 of the 25 most commonly prescribed drugs in older adults have anticholinergic effects. The cumulative effect of a number of drugs, or its total anticholinergic load, is probably more important. There are a number of scales available, such as the anticholinergic risk scale (ARS) that allocates each drug a number between 1 and 3 according to its anticholinergic potential, based on current data. Quetiapine, notably, is allocated 1 point.

Table 5.5 Anticholinergic activity of drugs expressed as ng/mL equivalent of atropine

Furosemide	0.22
Digoxin	0.25
Dyazide	0.08
Lanoxin	0.25
Hydrochlorothiazide	0.00
Propranolol, atenolol, metoprolol, timolol	0.00
Salicylic acid	0.00
Dipyridamole	0.11
Theophylline	0.44
Nitroglycerin	0.00
Insulin	0.00
Warfarin	0.12
Prednisolone	0.55
Alpha-methyldopa	0.00
Nifedipine	0.22
Isosorbide dinitrate	0.15
Ibuprofen	0.00
Codeine	0.11
Cimetidine	0.86
Diltiazem	0.00
Captopril	0.02
Ranitidine	0.22

Adapted with permission from Tune L *et al*. Anticholinergic effects of drugs commonly prescribed for the elderly: potential means for assessing risk of delirium. *American Journal of Psychiatry* 1992; 149: 1393–4.

Dopamine may be a precipitating factor, as shown in one study – but studies are lacking to identify its definite role (surprising as the drug is used to such a large extent).

Predisposing and/or precipitating factors

Environment

Do our patients need windows or clocks? Probably yes. Physicians have recognized that the quality of the environment influences the onset, severity and duration of delirium. An early and uncontrolled study suggested that sensory deprivation experienced by patients placed in windowless hospital rooms is associated with higher rates of delirium.

A study in the Netherlands comparing 55 patients nursed in an open ward with 75 patients in single rooms with daylight and additional measures to protect patients from unnecessary and excessive noise demonstrated a significant reduction in delirium of 0.5 days. This finding was not confirmed in a similar Canadian study in cardiac patients.

The association of delirium with visual impairment supports the idea of reduction of environmental stimuli as a risk factor. Patient care bundles targeted at minimizing predisposing risk factors involve frequent reorientation, provision of clocks, eyeglasses and hearing aids. These have been shown to reduce the incidence of delirium and improve short-term outcomes.

Studies on patient environment are difficult to do; a risk factor identified may well not be causal so interpretations of results need to be taken with care. An observational prospective study of 326 patients with delirium demonstrated an increase in the severity of delirium in those patients who underwent a number of room changes, those in the presence of a family member, those who did not have a clock, watch or reading glasses, and those with physical restraints. Note that physical medical restraints include urinary catheters and intravenous infusions.

But it is difficult to establish the confounding factors. Families are often called in when there is concern, the number of room changes may be related to the patient condition and some items may have been taken away because of the delirious state the patient is in.

Sleep

Lack of sleep affects cognitive functions; in 1845 a paper in the *American Journal of Insanity* quoted 'We wish we could impress upon all, the vast importance of securing sound and abundant sleep; if so, we should feel that we had done an immense good to our fellow-beings, not merely in preventing insanity, but other diseases also'. Sleep deprivation is often quoted as a risk factor for delirium and particularly in ICU where it is known that patients get very little if any 'normal' sleep at night. However, the relationship is still not well understood. Are patients not sleeping because they are delirious or delirious because they are not sleeping?

Delirium is up to ten times more likely to occur with severe sleep deprivation... but this is based on a subjective assessment of sleep deprivation. Patients with delirium seem to have less frequent and shorter REM (rapid eye movement) sleep episodes and longer REM latency than patients without delirium. The American Pain, Agitation and Delirium guidelines recommend promoting sleep in adult ICU patients by optimizing patients' environments, using strategies to control light and noise, clustering patient care activities, and decreasing stimuli at night to protect patients' sleep cycles. However, a review of 17 surgical studies did not establish sleep deprivation as a risk factor for delirium.

Benzodiazepines and opioid drugs influence the wake–sleep regulatory system and impact greatly on delirium. Conflicting studies report on the role of melatonin in critically ill patients.

The questions remain open: does delirium cause sleep deprivation? Or is delirium caused by altered sleep architecture or circadian rhythm desynchrony? Common sense would tell us that ensuring a good night's sleep for our patients will likely benefit brain function, but there is no evidence to back it up.

Exercise

Exercise is significantly protective against delirium in older medical patients. This includes self-reported regular exercise, reading books and newspapers, visiting relatives or friends.

Rehabilitation in critical care may utilize this! It is postulated that exercise increases grey and white matter volume in the prefrontal and temporal cortices (this is where age-related brain volume loss occurs); but it might just be that it increases cerebral blood flow – leading to a lower incidence of delirium.

Specific patient cohorts

Trauma patients

Predisposing and precipitating factors have been suggested in this population, with reduced Glasgow Coma Score (GCS), increased blood transfusion requirement and a higher Multiple Organ Failure Score being strong predictors for developing delirium. The Multiple Organ Failure Scale rates pulmonary, renal, cardiac and hepatic organ function. Surprisingly, age and trauma injury severity score did not contribute significantly to developing delirium when blood transfusions and the Multiple Organ Failure Score are taken into account.

In trauma patients, midazolam is associated with two- to threefold higher odds of transitioning into delirium each day, even after adjusting for covariates. Blood transfusions have been identified as an independent risk factor not only in trauma, but also in cardiac patients and after abdominal surgery.

Cardiac surgical patients

The risk of cerebral injury is increased in cardiac patients due to the underlying disease and unavoidable surgical techniques. Refreshingly, the risk factors for delirium after

cardiac surgery are generally consistent amongst studies
(contrary to many other fields as illustrated previously).
A previous stroke increases the risk of post-operative delirium
by up to eight times. Other risk factors include age over 65,
low albumin levels, preoperative atrial fibrillation and
depression. A possible preoperative prediction rule includes
four variables: prior stroke (1 point); low albumin (1 point);
depression (1 point); and Mini Mental State Examination
(MMSE) score of less than 23 (2 points) or between 24 and 27
(1 point). The delirium risk using this prediction score more
than quadrupled from the low-risk to the high-risk levels.

Prolonged duration of surgery and duration of
cardiopulmonary bypass have been identified as risk
factors for developing delirium. Both indicate increased
surgical complexity and risk. Preoperative cardiogenic shock,
low cardiac output and blood transfusions are also risk factors.
Low intraoperative lowest body temperature and intubation
time have been incriminated by others. It is still unknown if
avoiding cardiopulmonary bypass decreases the risk of
delirium. Studies on this do not compare like with like.

Persistent delirium

Delirium can persist beyond discharge, and identifying
modifiable factors is of the utmost importance for these patients.

One model is shown in Table 5.6. Another model
includes age over 84 years, cognitive impairment and
severe delirium, i.e. demonstrating eight of the diagnostic
symptoms.

Table 5.6 Independent risk factors for delirium at discharge

Risk factor	Adjusted OR (95% confidence interval)
Dementia, by diagnosis or modified Blessed Dementia Rating Scale > 4	2.3 (1.4–3.7)
Vision impairment	2.1 (1.3–3.2)
Activities of daily living impairment > 1	1.7 (1.2–3.0)
Charlson* Score > 4	1.7 (1.1–2.6)
Restraint use during delirirum	3.2 (1.9–5.2)

* *The Charlson Co-morbidity Index predicts the one-year mortality for a patient who may have a range of co-morbid conditions.*
Adapted with permission from Inouye SK *et al.* Risk factors for delirium at discharge: development and validation of a predictive model. *Archives of Internal Medicine* 2007; 167: 1406–13.

A preventative approach can simply include making sure the patient is using their spectacles! Physical restraints, not used a great deal in the UK but often discussed in the nursing literature and the coffee room, should not be used on older patients with delirium, as their use precipitates and prolongs delirium. Their use is often associated with increased agitation, immobility, functional decline, incontinence and pressure ulcers.

Key points

- ICU patients can have ten risk factors or more for developing delirium.
- It is important to establish whether a patient had cognitive impairment before admission.

- Early mobilization, visual aids and frequent reorientation may help modify delirium.
- Constantly review the need for additional drugs that may tip a patient into delirium.

FURTHER READING

Vanderbilt Delirium and Cognitive Impairment Study Group. www.icudelirium.org.

Elwood M. *Critical Appraisal of Epidemiological Studies and Clinical Trials*, 3rd edn. Oxford, Oxford University Press, 2007.

Inouye SK *et al.* A predictive model for delirium in hospitalized elderly medical patients based on admission characteristics. *Annals of Internal Medicine* 1993; 6: 474–81.

Chapter 6

Delirium in critical care: why is it important?

Introduction

Delirium is common, especially in vulnerable elderly patients or the seriously ill, it often goes unrecognized and the pathophysiology is still unclear. So what? This chapter is all about the 'so what', the adverse outcomes associated with delirium. Delirium is not benign.

Often the question is 'are patients dying with delirium or because of delirium?' This chapter will show that both statements are true.

Severity and duration of delirium

In 2013, the *New England Journal of Medicine* published a landmark study conducted in two centres in Nashville, Tennessee. Of 821 critically ill patients enrolled, cognitive deficits occurred in both older and younger patients and persisted, with 34% and 24% of all patients with assessments at 12 months that were similar to scores for patients with moderate traumatic brain injury and scores for patients with mild Alzheimer's disease, respectively. A longer duration of delirium was independently associated with worse global cognition at 3 and 12 months and worse executive function at 3 and 12 months. This was a particularly sick group of patients with a median Acute Physiology and Chronic Health Evaluation (APACHE) score of 25, and 30% had sepsis.

It appears that duration of delirium will have an impact on outcomes. Patients who develop subsyndromal delirium will have better outcomes than those who meet the full criteria, but worse than those with no delirium symptoms. This is true for both elderly medical patients and patients in intensive care. Those patients who recover from full-blown delirium before discharge will fare better than those who are admitted to rehabilitation hospitals with prevalent delirium.

This supports the idea that aggressively managing an episode of delirium in patients with a view to reducing the duration is beneficial. An obvious starting point is to screen all patients so the diagnosis can be made. In addition, persistence of symptoms in a patient up to discharge needs to be followed up.

Persistent delirium

Traditionally it has been thought that delirium is a temporary state and self-limiting even if it is not treated pharmacologically. However, as referred to in Chapter 2, some patients never recover completely and continue to demonstrate symptoms of delirium up to and following discharge.

It is thought that around half the patients with delirium on discharge from hospital will recover by 3 months, but the ones with persistent delirium lasting more than 3 months may never recover. Over 80% of these patients with persistent delirium are either in a nursing home or dead within 1 year.

Cause of death

Many patients die within months of a diagnosis of delirium and delirium remains an independent predictor of mortality. In one study, 41% of the patients who developed delirium died

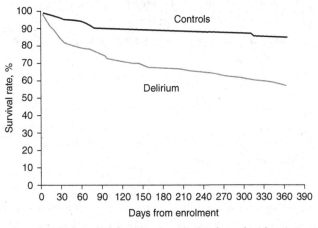

Figure 6.1 Impact of delirium on survival. Adapted with permission from McCusker J *et al*. Delirium predicts 12-month mortality. *Archives of Internal Medicine* 2002; 162: 457–63. Copyright © 2002 American Medical Association.

as opposed to 14% of those patients who didn't – these are crude mortality rates and there were a number of confounding factors. Nevertheless they reflect the significance of developing delirium.

After correction for all confounders i.e. severity of illness, co-morbidities, age and sex, the critically ill patient who becomes delirious is three times more likely to die within 6 months.

These patients do not die because they are sicker; they may very well die as a result of delirium. But why? We can speculate that in patients with sepsis, the acutely failing brain may help propagate the septic process by a loss of immune function modulation... Excess production of peripheral cytokines may go unchecked because of loss of central control... The lethargic patient fails to mobilize and subsequently develops chest infections, pressure sores and/or malnutrition... The agitated patient remains on sedation and ventilated for longer periods of time... Delirium is associated with falls...

Delirium is a strong independent marker of high risk of mortality not just in hospital, but for at least 11 months after admission. Among older medical patients delirium means a doubling of the risk of dying by 12 months.

Nothing, however, is simple in delirium. In the study quoted above, delirium had a particularly strong effect on mortality among patients **without** pre-existing dementia. In contrast, among patients **with** pre-existing dementia, there was a weaker, non-significant effect of delirium (and severity of delirium symptoms) on mortality. The explanation for this is not known, it may be down to the difficulty diagnosing delirium in the patient who has dementia, using surrogate assessments of dementia or that the delirium is a manifestation of an acute-on-chronic brain failure rather than due to a condition with further-reaching adverse consequences. Not enough is known.

Delirium has been shown to increase the risk of mortality in various patient groups recovering from surgery. Elderly patients who require intensive care post-operatively and develop delirium are more likely to die both in the short term (30 days) and the longer term (6 months).

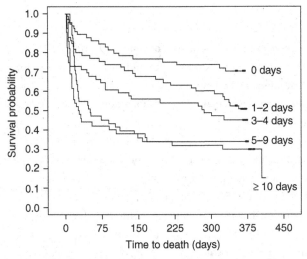

Figure 6.2 Kaplan–Meier survival curve for 1-year mortality post-intensive care unit (ICU) admission according to duration of delirium. Adapted with permission from Pisani MA *et al*. Days of delirium are associated with 1-year mortality in an older intensive care population. *American Journal of Respiratory and Critical Care Medicine* 2009; 180: 1092–7.

Hyperactive delirium appears to have a better prognosis than the subtle and easily missed hypoactive delirium. Patients with hyperactive delirium often have less severe physical illnesses than lethargic delirious patients. In addition, while agitated patients are more likely to fall, hypoactive patients are more prone to develop pressure sores and nosocomial infections. But there is a large variation in how clinicians manage motoric subtypes and it is difficult to identify if this in itself has an impact on outcome. It is easy to understand that patients who are a direct danger to themselves and staff because of delirium gain more attention from clinicians.

Each additional day an ICU patient spends in delirium is associated with a 10% increased risk of death.

Cognitive outcomes

Delirium is a precursor of poor cognitive outcomes in a variety of patient populations. It is believed that delirium could be one of the few preventable causes of long-term cognitive impairment.

There is a link between delirium and dementia, with a high incidence of delirium in patients with pre-existing dementia. Cognitive impairment has been consistently demonstrated to be a significant risk factor for delirium. Both dementia and delirium are associated with decreased cerebral metabolism, inflammation and cholinergic deficiency. Incident delirium has been shown to accelerate the trajectory of cognitive decline in hospitalized patients with Alzheimer's disease. Their cognitive function will decline at twice the expected rate in the year after hospitalization. This increased rate of decline is maintained for up to 5 years.

Evidence from clinical investigations regarding executive dysfunction suggests that delirium develops secondary to reduced blood flow in vulnerable subcortical structures, even in the absence of frank ischaemic injury. CT and MRI scans of the brains of critically ill patients in whom there is a concern about cerebral status are likely to show generalized brain atrophy, ventricular enlargement, white matter lesions and cortical and subcortical lesions. These patients are often unable to regain the independence they enjoyed before admission. The neuropsychological deficits may improve with time in some, but tend to be permanent in most cases.

The association between long-term cognitive impairment and episodes of delirium has been demonstrated, although causality and the potential for prevention remain elusive.

Although delirium may be a sign of emerging cognitive impairment, cognitive impairment subsequently experienced by a large number of patients with delirium is not solely or primarily related to pre-existing cognitive impairment.

It is likely that factors such as delirium subtype, duration, severity and aetiology may have implications for the degree of long-term cognitive impairment.

Functional recovery

Delirium is associated with worse functional outcomes. It is not necessarily an accelerated decline, but the patient recovers to a lower level of functional activity.

Functional status in patients is measured by asking patients (or surrogates) how well they manage with normal activities. Specific scoring systems exist such as the Activities of Daily Living (ADLs), Barthel Index or Katz Index that come up with a number representing how well a patient functions physically.

While the decline can be sustained, this is not always the case, and the degree of recovery depends on how completely the patient recovers from delirium, how long the episode lasted and whether it recurs. General medical patients who rapidly recover from an episode of delirium of less than 2 weeks can be expected over time to return to their normal level of functioning. It is suspected that severity and aetiology of the delirium may impact on rate and extent of recovery. Maybe a patient with a hospital drug-induced delirious episode of a couple of days recovers some basic physical functions more rapidly than if it was secondary to pneumonia, but maybe not.

Critically ill patients have worse functional outcomes if they have suffered delirium, many of whom will have had sepsis. Outside critical care, the worst functional outcomes associated

Table 6.1 The basic activities of daily living

- Personal hygiene
- Dressing and undressing
- Eating
- Transferring from bed to chair, and back
- Voluntarily controlling urinary and faecal discharge
- Elimination
- Moving around (as opposed to being bedridden)

Table 6.2 Katz Index of independence in activities of daily living

Activities (0 or 1 point)	Independence (1 point)	Dependence (0 point)
	NO supervision, direction or personal assistance	WITH supervision, direction, personal assistance or total care
BATHING	Bathes self completely or needs help in bathing only a single part of the body such as the back, genital area or disabled extremity	Needs help with bathing more than one part of the body, getting in or out of the tub or shower. Requires total bathing
DRESSING	Gets clothes from closets and drawers and puts on clothes and outer garments complete with fasteners. May have help tying shoes	Needs help with dressing self or needs to be completely dressed
TOILETING	Goes to toilet, gets on and off, arranges clothes, cleans genital area without help	Needs help transferring to the toilet, cleaning self or uses bedpan or commode
TRANSFERRING	Moves in and out of bed or chair unassisted. Mechanical transfer aids are acceptable	Needs help in moving from bed to chair or requires a complete transfer
CONTINENCE	Exercises complete self-control over urination and defecation	Is partially or totally incontinent of bowel or bladder
FEEDING	Gets food from plate into mouth without help. Preparation of food may be done by another person	Needs partial or total help with feeding or requires parenteral feeding

Score of 6 – High, patient is independent
Score of 0 – Low, patient is very dependent

Reprinted with permission from Katz S *et al.* Progress in development of the index of ADL. *Gerontologist* 1970; 10(1 Part 1): 20–30.

Table 6.3 Barthel Activity Daily Living Index

BOWELS	0 = Incontinent
	1 = Occasional accident (1 per week)
	2 = Continent
BLADDER	0 = Incontinent or catheterized and unable to manage
	1 = Occasional accident (max 1 × per 24 hours)
	2 = Continent for over 7 days
GROOMING	0 = Needs help
	1 = Independent, face, hair, teeth, shaving
TOILET USE	0 = Dependent
	1 = Needs some help but can do something
	2 = Independent (on and off, dressing, wiping)
FEEDING	0 = Unable
	1 = Needs help cutting, spreading butter etc.
	2 = Independent
TRANSFER	0 = Unable
	1 = Major help (1–2 people, physical)
	2 = Minor help (verbal or physical)
	3 = Independent
MOBILITY	0 = Immobile
	1 = Wheelchair independent including corners etc.
	2 = Walks with help of one person (verbal or physical)
	3 = Independent (but may use any aid, e.g. stick)
DRESSING	0 = Dependent
	1 = Needs help but can do half unaided
	2 = Independent
STAIRS	0 = Unable
	1 = Needs help (verbal, physical, carrying aid)
	2 = Independent up and down
BATHING	0 = Dependent
	1 = Independent

Reprinted with permission from Mahoney FI and Barthel DW. Functional evaluation: the Barthel Index. *Maryland State Medical Journal* 1965; 14: 61–5.

with delirium are seen in post-operative patients, particularly following admission for fractured neck of femur. But delirium could well be one of the main risk factors for falling... running in circles!

Apart from the duration, aetiology and severity of delirium, it is likely that pre-morbid level of function and functional reserve are important to how completely a patient can be rehabilitated. Patients who do not recover from their delirium, and have persistent delirium, will not recover functionally.

The fact that patients who recover quickly from delirium do well is important and should spur us on to screen for, and manage, delirium in critical care patients. If we can reduce the incidence and duration in our patients, this may improve functional outcomes. How well we function with day-to-day activities is a key determinant of quality of life.

Discharge: home or nursing home?

Is my patient able to return home after their critical illness?

Delirium has been shown to be a predictor of patients being discharged to an institution other than home in several patient groups including critically ill patients. As an indicator of a patient's outcome this paints a picture better than any scientific measure of function. This may be a consequence of new cognitive decline or, as previously explained, persistent delirium, either subsyndromal or full-blown. Delirium in patients with dementia, in particular, increases the likelihood of transfer to a long-term perhaps permanent care facility.

Psychological outcomes

Psychological outcomes after a stay in ICU include post-traumatic stress disorder (PTSD), anxiety and depression. PTSD requires the experience or witnessing of a severely traumatic and terrifying event. PTSD includes three symptom groups: re-experiencing, avoidance and physiological (such as sleeplessness). The symptoms cause significant distress and impair day-to-day functioning. One hypothesis is that PTSD may be triggered by delusional memories resulting from frightening psychotic experiences with delirium. PTSD is linked to the use of benzodiazepines and physical restraints, both of which are risk factors for developing delirium. It is noteworthy that a link between delirium and PTSD has not been established despite specific studies.

Patients who have no factual memories of their hospital stay clearly remember terrifying hallucinations, imagining they have to fight for their lives or their families' lives. Increasing evidence shows that even apparently calm patients with hypoactive delirium may be enduring frightening 'experiences' as part of their delirious state. Contrary to delirium, PTSD is more common in women and patients with pre-ICU psychopathology and poor coping skills.

Duration of stay

Not surprisingly delirium has been shown to be associated with longer duration of stay in ICUs; and in some ICU patients is the strongest independent determinant of duration of hospital stay (by as much as 10 days!).

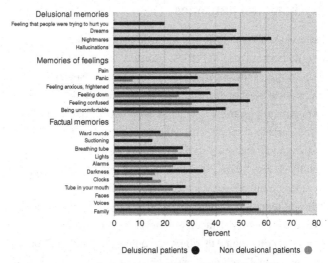

Figure 6.3 **Memories of patients in the ICU. Reprinted from Ringdal M *et al.*, Delusional memories from the intensive care unit – experienced by patients with physical trauma. *Intensive and Critical Care Nursing*, Vol. 22, Issue 6, pp. 346–54, Copyright 2006, with permission from Elsevier.**

The effect of delirium on duration of ICU stay is so important that it is independent of whether the patient is ventilated or not. The adverse outcomes associated with delirium will inevitably mean patients will be hospitalized for longer.

In the general medical population, post-admission delirium is a stronger predictor of duration of hospital stay than delirium on admission. This makes sense assuming that prevalent delirium might be part of the reasons for admission and is therefore managed more aggressively.

Collateral damage

Impact on families

Two thirds of relatives who visit patients on ICU have symptoms of anxiety or depression. More than 70% of spouses and nurses report severe stress related to delirium. Mean distress scores are significantly greater in fact for spouses/care givers than for staff or indeed the patients themselves. Not unexpectedly close family and friends find hyperactive delirium and poor functional status particularly upsetting. When talking to them, they are generally concerned that the change in behaviour is permanent, or that it reflects brain damage.

Impact on staff

Nursing staff caring for the hyperactive delirious patient often experience frustration and stress from trying to care for and treat the paranoid and violent patient who refuses to be comforted. Basic care and ensuring the safety of the patient is a real challenge. In critical care the danger is increased by the risks of disconnection of arterial lines, removal of central lines or accidental extubation.

Cost of delirium

It is a sobering thought that death is usually cheap in economic terms; however, longer duration of stay or poor functional recovery are expensive. In England, if mobilizing patients early decreases duration of ICU stay by 2 days, this could potentially save annually £13.4 million. The total burden of delirium on the US healthcare system has been estimated to be between 38 and 152 billion dollars.

While the short-term savings are known, or easy to calculate, establishing the cost of longer-term adverse outcomes is complex. Long-term cognitive impairment and decreased functional status cause a significant financial burden to society and families.

Key points

- Delirium has seriously bad outcomes.
- Delirium is an independent predictor of mortality.
- Delirium is a predictor of long-term cognitive impairment.
- ICU and hospital length of stay are increased with delirium.
- Delirium is expensive to society, and individuals.

FURTHER READING

www.icudelirium.org/outcomes.

James J *et al*. Research issues in the evaluation of cognitive impairment in intensive care unit survivors. *Intensive Care Medicine* 2004; 30: 2009–16.

Pandharipande PP *et al*. Long-term cognitive impairment after critical illness. *New England Journal of Medicine* 2013; 369: 1306–16.

Chapter 7

Delirium in critical care: monitoring tools

Introduction

How to detect delirium in the critically ill patients even when they are sedated? Don't worry, it is easy... but only if you look for it. Most patients present with hypoactive delirium, a lethargic apparently co-operative patient; but just scratch the surface and you will find an inattentive patient with altered mental status and disorganized thinking.

A 69-year-old patient was recovering from an infection of his urinary tract that had led to major sepsis. He still required haemofiltration intermittently and consequently was only mobilizing slowly. He appeared as a quiet and co-operative patient, but was extremely reluctant to eat. The clinicians and dietician made sure he was not constipated, and prescribed nutritional supplements while encouraging him to eat. The team suspected he was depressed. It was only after discharge, when he was seen in the follow-up clinic, that he told the consultant that he had been frightened whilst on the unit, believing that the staff were feeding him up so they could eat him for Christmas! The ICU staff had no idea.

Delirium screening is recommended routinely for all critically ill patients by the UK National Institute for Health and Care Excellence (NICE) and the American College of

Critical Care Medicine. It doesn't need any equipment, there is no risk to the patient and takes around 2 minutes (if that) ... how many interventions in ICU are so quick and easy?

Clinical monitoring of the brain

Delirium is a clinical syndrome, and the diagnosis is made at the bedside. In the past we thought in order to assess a patient's mental status it was enough to ask them to follow a simple command, usually to put their tongue out; or even just ask them if they were comfortable.

However, delirious patients can often follow direct commands and will mostly give an affirmative answer to any question. Today screening tools are needed to ensure adequate assessment and must be used routinely to ensure that a patient's examination is complete.

Diagnosing delirium requires a combination of a positive result with a screening tool and a high index of clinical suspicion. Screening is important because delirium can assume so many forms with variable and fluctuating clinical signs. In intensive care this is further compounded by the fact that our patients are often sedated and intubated.

If the screening test is positive, the clinician will seek further evidence of precipitating risk factor(s) such as signs of a new infection or the administration of specific drugs.

Monitoring the brain involves two steps

Consciousness is awareness of self and of the environment. Simplistically it has two aspects: **arousal**, which is the state of wakefulness, and **content of cognition**, which is the sum of mental activities, including memory, calculation, sensory awareness and visuospatial skills.

The **first step** of monitoring the brain is to assess the *level of consciousness or arousal*. Sedation scores are routinely used

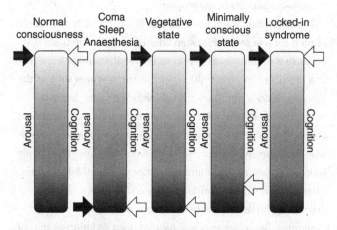

Figure 7.1 Graphical representation of the two components of consciousness (arousal and cognition) and their alterations in coma, the vegetative state, the minimally conscious state and in the locked-in syndrome. Reprinted from the *Lancet Neurology* volume 3, Issue 9, Laureys S *et al*. Brain function in coma, vegetative state, and related disorder. pp. 537–46, Copyright 2004, with permission from Elsevier.

in most ICUs and clinicians are familiar with using level of consciousness as a vital sign (how awake is my patient?).

The **second step** is a test of *mental status, the content of brain function.* Is my patient able to make sense of the environment? There are an increasing number of senior clinicians who believe mental status should be the sixth vital sign.

Sedation scores (or arousal scales)

Sedation scores are not delirium screening tools – even the ones with agitation in their name.

The Richmond Agitation-Sedation Scale, RASS, is commonly quoted for use as the first step when screening the brain because it differentiates response to verbal stimulus from that to a physical stimulus, unlike other sedation scores such as the Ramsay. It does not matter which sedation score a unit is using, the important point is that an assessment of wakefulness is done. In order to screen for mental status, you need a patient who is responsive, preferably to a verbal stimulus. The deeply sedated or comatose patient cannot be screened for delirium. These patients unarousable to voice (RASS −4 or −5) are classed as 'unable to assess' and have consistently poorer outcomes. Some patients will require deep sedation as part of the management of their critical illness.

The dangers of over-sedation are well known; the benefits of daily wake-ups proven. Patients should only be maintained in deep sedation for as long as it is clinically indicated, e.g. the difficult-to-ventilate asthmatic.

Content of cognition or mental status

The expressions 'clouding of consciousness' or 'altered sensorium', often used when describing delirium, actually refer more to a patient's cognition – awareness of self, surroundings and ability to make sense of this – than level of arousal. It is considerably more difficult to test, even difficult to describe! A medical dictionary would define it: 'a disturbance of consciousness in which a patient cannot think clearly and has difficulty paying attention to what is happening or what is being said'. Inattention means not only the loss of ability to focus and pay attention but also the inability to shift attention. So when using a test for inattention such as asking them to squeeze only on the 'A's' in a 10-letter sequence, the delirious patient may squeeze and then not let go until asked to.

To understand mental status, examine a patient non-intubated, see if the patient is easily distracted or over-absorbed in a task (for example rearranging the sheet), then use the reverse test digit span (a simple tool looking for inattention: ask a patient to repeat an increasing series of random numbers backwards, e.g. 8, 4, 3 then 8, 4, 3, 7 and so on – they should be able to remember at least five numbers, fewer than that indicates inattention). Next, ask the patient to 'describe their medical problems' and establish if they can organize their thoughts in a coherent way. End by asking them if they feel unsafe or are having hallucinations.

Table 7.1 Commonly used sedation scales in adults

Ramsay Scale

1   Anxious and agitated or restless or both
2   Co-operative, orientated and tranquil
3   Responding to commands only
4   Brisk response to light glabellar tap
5   Sluggish response to light glabellar tap
6   No response to light glabellar tap

Motor Activity Assessment Scale MAAS

0   Unresponsive
1   Responsive only to noxious stimuli
2   Responsive to touch or when name is spoken loudly
3   Calm and co-operative
4   Restless and co-operative
5   Agitated
6   Dangerously agitated, unco-operative

Richmond Agitation-Sedation Scale RASS

+4   Combative – Overtly combative, violent, immediate danger to staff
+3   Very agitated – Pulls or removes tube(s) or catheter(s), aggressive
+2   Agitated – Frequent non-purposeful movement, fights ventilator
+1   Restless – Anxious, but movements not aggressive or vigorous
0   Alert and calm
−1   Drowsy – Not fully alert, but has sustained awakening (eye opening/eye contact) to voice (> 10 sec)
−2   Light sedation – Briefly awakens with eye contact to voice (< 10 sec)
−3   Moderate sedation – Movement or eye opening to voice (but no eye contact)
−4   Deep sedation – No response to voice, but movement or eye opening to physical stimulation*
−5   Non arousable – No response to voice or physical stimulation

---

* *Physical stimulation: shaking and/or rubbing sternum.*

Reprinted with permission from Ramsay M *et al.* Controlled sedation with alphaxalone-alphadolone. *British Medical Journal* 1974; 2: 656–9; Devlin JW *et al.* Motor Activity Assessment Scale: a valid and reliable sedation scale for use with mechanically ventilated patients in an adult surgical intensive care unit. *Critical Care Medicine* 1999; 27: 1271–5; Sessler CN *et al.* The Richmond Agitation-Sedation Scale: validity and reliability in adult intensive care unit patients. *American Journal of Respiratory and Critical Care Medicine* 2002; 166: 1338–44.

When assessing a patient's mental status do the Confusion Assessment Method for the ICU (CAM-ICU) (see later in this chapter), but also talk with patients, observe them critically and listen.

Clinical screening tools

The Holy Grail of delirium science is a reliable, reproducible and easy-to-use screening tool. Clinicians are used to rates and pressures and handle numbers. Intensive care clinicians in particular are reliant on electronic monitors and can find assessment of mental status a challenge. Two clinicians taking a pulse rate are going to agree the vast majority of the time. Similarly with sedation scores, good inter-rater reliability is expected when assessing whether a patient responds to a verbal stimulus or a physical stimulus. Deciding whether a patient is easily distracted (inattention) or has a perceptual disturbance requires time and practice. The difficulty has been solved by tools that have been developed specifically for critically ill patients to be used at the bedside.

The emphasis in defining delirium has shifted over the years from an extensive list of symptoms to the two essential concepts of **disordered attention** (arousal) and **cognition**, while continuing to recognize the importance of acute onset and organic aetiology.

The ideal delirium assessment tool will reliably evaluate the primary components of delirium, i.e. consciousness, inattention, disorganized thinking and fluctuating course; be valid in a diverse critical care population; be completed quickly and easily; and will not require extra equipment or the presence of psychiatric personnel.

Delirium assessment: variety of tools

Several tools are used in hospital patients but only four have been validated in critically ill patients against the gold standard (i.e. DSM-IV criteria and features of delirium). A number of instruments have been developed to assess delirium in clinical practice and for research purposes. They have different formats, such as algorithms, short interviews and scales. Some are specifically designed for diagnosing the presence of delirium, others to describe the symptoms and rate their severity. Clinicians should ensure that the tool they use is validated for their type of patients.

Developing a screening tool for ICU

The first delirium screening tool validated for ICU patients was the Cognitive Test for Delirium, but it is not generally used. It was designed to assess for a number of symptoms of delirium using five subtests with non-verbal responses. The test administration takes 10 to 15 minutes for each patient. An abbreviated Cognitive Test for Delirium was subsequently developed as a more practical version although not validated – this test is the same as the part screening for inattention using picture recognition as in the CAM-ICU (see later in this chapter).

The CAM-ICU and the Intensive Care Delirium Screening Checklist (ICDSC) were both published in 2001. These days, most units screening ICU patients for delirium will use one of these two tests. They were both developed and validated as clinical tools to be used at the bedside for the routine screening and diagnosis of delirium in ICU patients. Currently, individual units decide which test to use based on local preferences.

The Nursing Delirium Scale (Nu-DESC) was first described in 2005 and subsequently used to screen for post-operative delirium in non-ventilated patients. A validation study suggesting it as an alternative to CAM-ICU in non-ventilated patients was published in 2010 [9].

The Neelon and Champagne (NEECHAM) scale was assessed for use in ICU patients (2006). This nursing observation scale has not so far been proved to be useful in intubated patients.

Mini Mental State Examination (MMSE)

The MMSE is a global test of cognition and not a stand-alone delirium screening tool. Outside of critical care the MMSE has become one of the most frequently used neuropsychological tests in the clinical evaluation of delirium. It was originally conceived as a short, 5 to 10 minutes, practical clinical instrument to distinguish functional from organic mental status impairment. It includes 11 simple questions, including 2 with written answers, to give a score depending on correct responses of a maximum of 30 and a cut-off for cognitive impairment of 24. The questions test orientation to time and space, instantaneous recall, short-term memory, serial subtractions or reverse spelling (the word world), constructional capacity and use of language. It is fairly self-explanatory and as such can be administered by anyone, clinician or non-clinician. As with all such tests there is need for caution when interpreting small changes, especially if the testers are different.

The current version of the MMSE, which was previously freely available, is now owned by Psychological Assessment Resources (PAR). Despite the many free versions of the test that are available on the internet, the official version is copyrighted and PAR must be paid for every single use. The enforcement of copyright with resulting lawsuits has led to researchers and clinicians looking for alternatives when assessing cognition, e.g. Montreal Cognitive Assessment (MOCA), which is more able to detect mild cognitive impairment and is free for clinical and educational use although permission is needed for use in research projects (see Figure 7.2).

Confusion Assessment Method (CAM)

The Confusion Assessment Method has been in use since 1990. It is an easy-to-administer instrument that has gained the approval of the British Geriatrics Society. It involves an

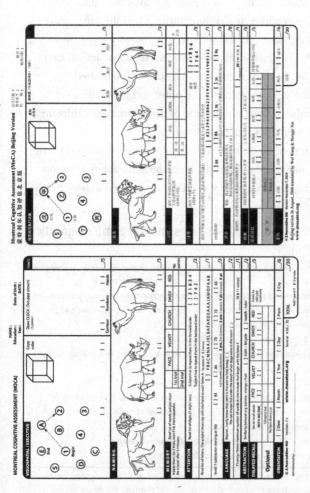

Figure 7.2 The Montreal Cognitive Assessment test. Image downloaded from www.mocatest. org, where the test is freely available in multiple languages. Illustration presents the English and Chinese versions. Copyright Z. Nasreddine MD. Reproduced with permission.

interview with the patient to look for the presence or absence of nine clinical features of delirium: acute onset and fluctuating course; inattention; disorganized thinking; altered level of consciousness; disorientation; memory impairment; perceptual disturbance; abnormal psychomotor activity and altered sleep–wake cycle. The diagnosis is established according to four criteria: acute onset and fluctuating symptoms with inattention; and either disorganized thinking and/or altered level of consciousness.

When used by trained health professionals it performs well against psychiatric diagnosis. It can be administered by non-clinicians, following training, and be completed in less than 5

Table 7.2 The Confusion Assessment Method diagnostic algorithm

Feature 1	**Acute onset and fluctuating course**

Is there evidence of an acute change in mental status from the patient's baseline? Did the (abnormal) behaviour fluctuate during the day, i.e. come and go, or increase and decrease in severity?

Feature 2	**Inattention**

Did the patient have difficulty focusing attention, e.g. being easily distractable, or having difficulty keeping track of what was being said?

Feature 3	**Disorganized thinking**

Was the patient's thinking disorganized or incoherent, such as rambling or irrelevant conversation, unclear or illogical flow of ideas, or unpredictable switching from subject to subject?

Feature 4	**Altered level of consciousness**

Anything other than alert, i.e. hyperalert or lethargic

Adapted with permission from Inouye SK *et al*. Clarifying confusion: the confusion assessment method. A new method for detection of delirium. *Annals of Internal Medicine* 1990; 113: 941–8.

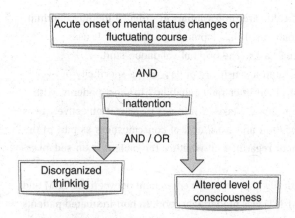

Figure 7.3 Schematic overview of the four criteria of the Confusion Assessment Method.

minutes. The MMSE, an instrument to evaluate cognitive function, is often used with the CAM, in which case the assessment will take 10 to 15 minutes.

The CAM is widely used although in some reports it does not always perform as well with regard to sensitivity or specificity as the initial study demonstrated. It is however, once the ongoing training issues are addressed, an invaluable tool to assist in the diagnosis of the delirious patient.

Confusion Assessment Method for the ICU (CAM-ICU)

The Confusion Assessment Method for the ICU (CAM-ICU) was developed as a brief, accurate and reliable instrument for use by healthcare professionals in order to identify delirium in ICU patients. It is adapted from the CAM. It uses non-verbal tasks. The original validation studies demonstrated a sensitivity of 93% and a specificity of over 98%, with high inter-rater reliability. In most patients, with practice it literally takes 2 minutes or less. It objectively tests for inattention and uses level of consciousness as part of the assessment regardless of whether the patient is on sedatives or not.

In critically ill patients the agreement between the CAM and the CAM-ICU was moderately good. In non-intubated patients with good verbal capabilities the CAM-ICU has high specificity but is less sensitive at detecting delirium than the CAM with the MMSE – but it can be applied much more quickly, i.e. 30 seconds to 2 minutes maximum. The Brief Confusion Assessment Method (b-CAM) has been developed to improve the sensitivity of the CAM-ICU in non-intubated patients with the addition of the request to spell LUNCH backwards and to say the months of the year backwards to July.

With the CAM-ICU, the patient is initially assessed for altered or fluctuating mental status, inattention is tested using a 10-letter sequence where the patient is required to squeeze the clinician's hand only when the letter A is stated. The patient is then assessed for disorganized thinking by their ability to answer four simple yes/no questions and a command, and finally for reduced level of consciousness. Patients are defined as delirious if altered mental status and inattention are present with disorganized thinking and/or reduced level of consciousness. This test can be performed on

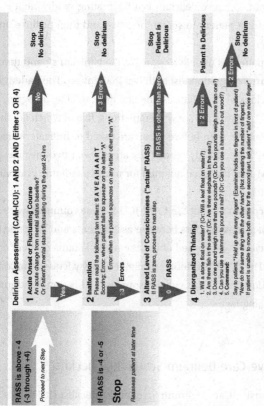

Confusion Assessment Method in the ICU

RASS is above - 4
(-3 through +4)
Proceed to next Step

If RASS is -4 or -5
Stop
Reassess patient at later time

Delirium Assessment (CAM-ICU): 1 AND 2 AND (Either 3 OR 4)

1 Acute Onset or Fluctuating Course
An acute change from mental status baseline?
Or Patient's mental status fluctuating during the past 24 hrs

→ No → **Stop No delirium**

↑ Yes

2 Inattention
Please read the following ten letters: S A V E A H A A R T
Scoring: Error: when patient fails to squeeze on the letter "A"
Error: when the patient squeezes on any letter other than "A"

→ < 3 Errors → **Stop No delirium**

↑ ≥3 Errors

3 Altered Level of Consciousness ("actual" RASS)
If RASS is other than zero, proceed to next step

→ If RASS is other than zero → **Stop Patient is Delirious**

↑ 0 RASS

4 Disorganized Thinking
1. Will a stone float on water? (Or: Will a leaf float on water?)
2. Are there fish in the sea? (Or: Are there elephants in the sea?)
3. Does one pound weigh more than two pounds? (Or: Do two pounds weigh more than one?)
4. Can you use a hammer to pound a nail? (Or: Can you use a hammer to cut wood?)
5. Command:
Say to patient: "Hold up this many fingers" (Examiner holds two fingers in front of patient)
"Now do the same thing with the other hand" (Not repeating the number of fingers).
If patient is unable to move both arms for the second part, ask patient "add one more finger"

→ ≥ 2 Errors → **Patient is Delirious**

→ < 2 Errors → **Stop No delirium**

Figure 7.4 Confusion Assessment Method in the ICU to detect delirium with its four criteria: acute onset and fluctuating symptoms with inattention; and either disorganized thinking and/or altered level of consciousness. (CAM-ICU, Copyright by E. Wesley Ely, MD, MPH.)

any patient who will open their eyes and keep their eyes open to a verbal stimulus, usually saying their name. Patients either screen positive or negative and it is a point-in-time assessment. Because delirium is a fluctuating syndrome it is possible for a patient to screen negative and then positive an hour later.

If the patient is unable to squeeze the clinician's hand there is a picture recognition test to detect inattention. The patient is asked to look at five pictures one at a time, a table, a dagger, a cat, etc. They are then shown ten pictures, five of which are the ones they have seen before. They are asked to indicate which ones they have already seen. They are allowed two mistakes. The CAM-ICU has been adapted for use in paediatric critically ill patients.

We recommend that the CAM-ICU is done routinely twice a shift with at least 4 hours between assessments and repeated if the clinician is concerned about the mental status of their patient. The CAM-ICU tool is available at www.icudelirium.org for free download, with video resources, and is translated into over 25 languages.

Intensive Care Delirium Screening Checklist

The Intensive Care Delirium Screening Checklist (ICDSC) is a screening checklist of eight items: altered level of consciousness; inattention; disorientation; hallucinations or delusions; psychomotor agitation or retardation; inappropriate mood or speech; sleep–wake cycle disturbance and symptom fluctuation. It is recorded over a period of time, and utilizes as many elements as possible from routinely collected data. There is a degree of subjective interpretation, e.g. for inattention. If a patient demonstrates an item at any time they get a score of 1 point, for a maximum score of 8. A score of 4 points or more equates with delirium. If a patient is on sedative drugs the altered level of consciousness is not included. The ICDSC has been demonstrated to detect subsyndromal delirium as opposed to the CAM-ICU where a patient can have hallucinations yet still screen negative. A positive score of less than 4 equates with subsyndromal delirium. Subsyndromal delirium in critically ill patients has been associated with longer ICU stay and higher level of care after ICU discharge compared with patients who did not develop delirium. This test has a reported sensitivity of 99% and a specificity of 64%.

The ICDSC is a checklist of information gathered over a shift, generally without the need for an additional test. If the nurse observes a feature (e.g. a patient reaching out to grab an unseen object, presumably hallucinating), this is ticked off as present during the shift. Inattention is assessed subjectively by observing signs such as being easily distracted or difficulty following commands.

If the patient is on sedative drugs, the ICDSC asks the bedside nurse to judge whether inattention or decreased psychomotor activity is due to recent sedation, and not to score this as a positive delirium symptom. Also remember level of consciousness does not count if the patient is on sedation.

Table 7.3 Intensive Care Delirium Screening Checklist

Altered level of consciousness		
	A – No response	Stop*
	B – Response to intense and repeated stimulation (loud voice and pain)	Stop*
	C – Response to mild to moderate stimulation	1
	D – Normal wakefulness	0
	E – Exaggerated response to normal stimulation	1
*** If A or B, do not complete patient evaluation**		
Inattention		0 or 1
Disorientation		0 or 1
Hallucination – delusion – psychosis		0 or 1
Psychomotor agitation or retardation		0 or 1
Inappropriate speech or mood		0 or 1
Sleep/wake cycle disturbance		0 or 1
Symptom fluctuation		0 or 1

Reprinted with kind permission from Springer Science+Business Media. Bergeron *et al*. Intensive Care Delirium Screening Checklist: evaluation of a new screening tool. *Intensive Care Medicine* 2001; 27(5): 859–64.

Comparing CAM-ICU and ICDSC

In a sedated patient, the observer using the ICDSC will be asked to discard inattention if they believe it is due to sedation; while the CAM-ICU considers inattention to be a positive feature for delirium whether the patient is sedated or not. In addition, reduced level of consciousness will not score 1 on the ICDSC if a patient is sedated.

The two scoring systems have a high level of agreement. One study observed 126 patients and compared these screening tests against the gold standard (DSM-IV criteria). Thirty-four per cent of the patients were delirious when assessed with the DSM-IV criteria. Using the CAM-ICU, 29% were flagged as delirious, and most were the same patients (sensitivity of 64% and specificity of 88%); using the ICDSC, 19% were delirious (sensitivity of 43% and specificity of 95%). Rather good when considering that the clinicians using judgement only detected fewer than a third of patients who were DSM-IV delirious.

The latest Clinical Practice Guidelines from the American College of Critical Care Medicine state that the CAM-ICU and the ICDSC are the most valid and reliable monitoring tools for delirium in adult ICU patients. Currently, which one a unit uses routinely to assess patients depends on local preferences. It is important that the staff are confident in its use. What is not in doubt is that a screening tool is needed in order to detect delirium in critically ill patients.

NEECHAM scale

The Neelon and Champagne (NEECHAM) scale for non-intubated critically ill patients is a nine-item scale separated into three categories: ability to process information, behaviour and physiological condition. Patients are categorized according to 'degrees of confusion' ranging from non-delirious through to at risk, early to mild confusion and moderate to severe, i.e. delirious. This test is not yet considered user-friendly for intubated patients.

Nurses have expressed doubts using 'appearance' in patients who are unable to dress themselves, posture in patients who may have polyneuropathy and physiological parameters as indicators of delirium in patients on ventilators.

The incidence of delirium in non-intubated patients obtained with the NEECHAM scoring test is similar to the one obtained with the CAM-ICU.

Table 7.4 NEECHAM Confusion Scale

Level 1 – Processing

Attention – Attention – Alertness – Responsiveness

Full attentiveness/alertness	4
Short or hyper attention/alertness	3
Attention/alertness inconsistent or inappropriate	2
Attention/alertness disturbed	1
Arousal/responsiveness depressed	0

Command – Recognition – Interpretation – Action

Able to follow a complex command	5
Slowed complex command response	4
Able to follow a single command	3
Unable to follow direct command	2
Unable to follow visual guided command	1
Hypoactive, lethargic	0

Orientation – Orientation – Short-Term Memory – Thought/Speech Content

Oriented to time, place and person	5
Oriented to person and place	4
Orientation inconsistent	3
Disoriented and memory/recall disturbed	2
Disoriented, disturbed recognition	1
Processing of stimuli depressed	0

Level 2 – Behaviour

Appearance

Controls posture, maintains appearance, hygiene	2
Either posture or appearance disturbed	1
Both posture and appearance abnormal	0

Table 7.4 (cont.)

Motor	
Normal motor behaviour	4
Motor behaviour slowed or hyperactive	3
Motor movement disturbed	2
Inappropriate, disruptive movements	1
Motor movement depressed	0
Verbal	
Initiates speech appropriately	4
Limited speech initiation	3
Inappropriate speech	2
Speech/sound disturbed	1
Abnormal sounds	0
Level 3 – Physiological control	
Physiological measurements	
Systolic and diastolic blood pressure, heart rate, temperature, respiration rate within normal range with regular pulse	2
Any one of the above in abnormal range	1
Two or more in abnormal range	0
Oxygen therapy	
Not prescribed	0
Prescribed but not on	1
Prescribed and on	2
Oxygen saturation stability	
O_2 sat in normal range (93 or above)	2
O_2 sat 90 to 92 or is receiving oxygen	1
O_2 sat below 90	0
Urinary continence	
Maintains bladder control	2
Incontinent of urine in last 24 hours or has condom catheter in place	1
Incontinent now or has indwelling or intermittent catheter or is anuric	0

Adapted with permission from Neelon VJ *et al.* The NEECHAM Confusion Scale: construction, validation and clinical testing. *Nursing Research* 1996; 45(6): 324–30.

Table 7.5 Nursing Delirium Scale (Nu-DESC) – score 1 if required – a score of 2 is positive for delirium

	Midnight to 8 am	8 am to 4 pm	4 pm to midnight
1. Disorientation			
Verbal or behavioural manifestation of not being orientated to time or place or misperceiving persons in the environment			
2. Inappropriate behaviour			
Behaviour inappropriate to place and/or for the person; e.g. pulling at tubes or dressings, attempting to get out of bed when that is contraindicated and the like			
3. Inappropriate communication			
Communication inappropriate to place and/or for the person; e.g. incoherence, non-communicativeness, nonsensical or unintelligible speech			
4. Illusions/hallucinations			
Seeing or hearing things that are not there; distortions of visual objects			
5. Psychomotor retardation			
Delayed responsiveness, few or no spontaneous actions/words; e.g. when the patient is prodded, reaction is deferred and/or the patient is unarousable			
Total score			

Adapted with permission from Gaudreau JD *et al.* Fast, systematic and continuous delirium assessment in hospitalized patients: the Nursing Delirium Screening Scale. *Journal of Pain and Symptom Management* 2005; 29: 368–75.

The Nursing Delirium Scale (Nu-DESC)

The Nursing Delirium Scale is a five-item scale screening specifically for psychomotor retardation as well as disorientation, inappropriate behaviour or communication and hallucinations. As with the ICDSC it relies for the most part on observation rather than patient interaction – a score of 2 or more is positive for delirium. It has a comparable sensitivity to CAM-ICU but is not as specific according to DSM-IV criteria. Because it is a graded scale it is likely to be useful in detecting subsyndromal delirium.

Screening patients using the CAM-ICU

The comatose unresponsive patient

On approaching a patient, establish a response by calling out their name. If they do not respond, try a light physical stimulus while calling their name. If they do not awaken, or open their eyes and immediately close them, they cannot be assessed for delirium at that time – review the clinical needs of the patient regarding sedation. If they do not need to be deeply sedated, decide a target, e.g. RASS –1, and stop sedation until they reach this and can be assessed. In order to maintain this target once they are awake restart the sedation at half the original rate and then titrate for a steady state. Obviously analgesic requirements will need to be specifically addressed.

The awake unresponsive patient

On a patient opening their eyes the tester should introduce themselves and explain to the patient that they are going to test their thinking. Then ask the patient to squeeze your hand. If the patient does nothing and there is no reason to believe they are physically incapable of squeezing a hand, this patient has severe inattention and screens positive. If they are unable to use their hands then you could ask them to nod their head or even blink or use the picture recognition test described earlier in this chapter. If a patient cannot comprehend commands such as 'nod your head' or 'squeeze my hand' in everyday life they cannot be assessed. Note that a diagnosis of dementia on its own does not preclude assessment.

The awake responsive patient

Once a patient has squeezed your hand go on to explain that you are going to say ten letters and you want them to squeeze only on the letter A, repeat this. Then use the sequence SAVE A HAART making sure you leave enough time between letters for a response. They are allowed two mistakes (squeezing on a non-A or not on an A) before you can say they are inattentive. If they have two or fewer mistakes they are not inattentive and so are not delirious, they are CAM-ICU negative. The test is complete.

The inattentive responsive patient

Commonly, inattentive patients will either: (1) not squeeze your hand at all on any letters; or (2) squeeze on every letter; or (3) start off well but make mistakes towards the last four or five letters. Patients who do not squeeze at all are so inattentive that although they are capable of following a direct command, they are unable to follow simple instructions which have to be remembered for more than a few seconds.

More than two mistakes? Go on and assess for a reduced level of consciousness and/or disorganized thinking.

Disorganized thinking is established in two parts. First ask the patient to follow a simple command. Show the patient two raised fingers and ask them to raise the same number. Once they do this ask them to do the same with their other hand or to raise one more. Doing this involves organizing thoughts. The patient who is unable to do this may look at one hand and then the other without being able to figure out what to do!

Secondly ask four simple yes/no questions (there are two sets provided) such as 'are there fish in the sea?' and 'will a stone float on water?' The new tester may feel self-conscious asking these questions but remember you have already established this patient has inattention. You are not asking a patient who has normal thought processes. Classically, the patient who is delirious will answer yes to all the questions asked of them. Of the one command and four questions the patient is allowed to get one wrong. More than one wrong or a reduced level of consciousness and the patient is CAM-ICU positive and the clinician needs to decide how to manage this (how to manage these patients is explained in Chapters 8 and 9).

When we are unable to assess

Apart from unresponsive patients, other patients who are difficult to assess include patients who do not speak the local language and cannot understand, patients who have suffered strokes with expressive or receptive dysphasia, those with extensive facial or limb trauma and quadriplegic patients. While it can be difficult to assess these patients, with imagination, effort and assistance from relatives it can often be done.

When the screening is negative but the patient is hallucinating

After introducing yourself to your patient and explaining the test you will often find the patients who are not delirious concentrate hard on doing it well. The patient is often aware that their powers of concentration are not good and may have experienced some perceptual disturbances, usually visual hallucinations, so are keen to have their thinking tested. Also it is an interaction they seem to welcome; instead of doing something to them such as taking blood or giving drugs we are asking for a response and involving them in a two-way exchange. Similarly relatives are always concerned about the cognitive status of their loved ones and are reassured we are monitoring this.

The CAM-ICU can be negative when a patient has hallucinations. Perceptual disturbances are a symptom of delirium; however, their presence is not required for the diagnosis. The patient who has hallucinations and who is CAM-ICU negative may be suffering from subsyndromal delirium which is not detected by the CAM-ICU. But these patients may become CAM-ICU positive later and it is advisable to repeat the CAM-ICU more frequently than once a shift.

Additional note: if a patient tells you about hallucinations it is important to talk to them about how common they are in critically ill patients, that they are part of the illness, are temporary and while often quite terrifying and vivid, they are ultimately tricks of the mind. If the patient is concerned about strong delusional memories they may need referring to a psychiatrist because of the association between delusional memories, rather than episodes of delirium, and post-traumatic stress syndrome.

Screening patients using the ICDSC

At the start of a clinical shift, a new copy of the checklist is attached to the daily chart.

The level of consciousness is assessed first and if a patient is unrousable or only responsive to a painful stimulus throughout the shift, the patient cannot be assessed.

If the patient is responsive to touch or lighter, up to agitated, the nurse will score 1.

Throughout the shift, signs of delirium will be marked as present at the time they are apparent by inserting a 1 in the corresponding section:

Inattention: Does the patient have difficulty following a conversation or an instruction? Are they easily distracted by an external stimulus, e.g. do they follow with their eyes? Once they start something, are they able to turn to another task, e.g. once they squeeze your hand, do they let go?

Disorientation: Believing they are somewhere else in time or space, failing to recognize the nurse who looked after them the day before?

Hallucinations or delusions: Often obvious or can be deduced from behaviour, also ask patient specifically.

Psychomotor agitation or retardation: Constantly restless or noticeably still, or never shifting position or moving limbs.

Inappropriate speech or mood: Inappropriate, disorganized or incoherent speech, flat affect, emotionally labile, overly demanding.

Sleep–wake cycle disturbance: Not sleeping at night or apparently not at all in a 24-hour period or asleep most of the time.

Symptom fluctuation: Changes in above items within or between shifts.

A total score is calculated at the end of a shift and if equal or above 4, it indicates delirium. The score does not relate to the severity.

Implementing delirium screening

Once clinicians appreciate the importance of screening for delirium in critically ill patients the next step is to start it in their own practice and make it routine in their own units. As with any change implementation, however worthy, this can be a significant challenge. It does require application and commitment.

Constraints

In CAM-ICU implementation studies, it has been shown that once routine screening is in place nurses will often do the delirium assessment more than once a shift. They believe it is of benefit to the patient. There will only be any benefit if actions are taken on the result of the evaluation.

When asked about the constraints to screening the most frequently quoted by nurses were lack of time and medical staff buy-in. The assessment takes on average 2 minutes once a shift, but this can be an issue when countless interventions are all battling for time.

Medical engagement is required to ensure that patients receive attention and any appropriate treatment when scored positive. The nurse will see little point in finding out whether a patient is CAM-ICU positive or scores more than 4 on the ICDSC if this is ignored.

Some intensivists believe it is not necessary to screen as treatment has not been proven to improve outcomes. Most

ICU patients with delirium are therefore left untreated, because it is usually undiagnosed or no treatment is made available. Importantly, ICU delirium can be the first sign of a new infection, and the astute clinician will integrate this information when assessing a patient.

A survey of doctors in training concluded that it is a lack of knowledge in the diagnosis and management of delirium that explains its under-recognition, rather than a lack of awareness of its high prevalence and clinical significance.

An essential part of an implementation programme is deciding a course of action once it is clear a patient is delirious. Failure to take delirium seriously and to take action is often a result of lack of knowledge and frequent changes of resident medical staff can create ongoing problems for the bedside nurse.

A number of resources are available on the internet to help implement delirium screening (see www.icudelirium.org and www.icudelirium.co.uk).

Finally, the brain roadmap!

The clinician should use the brain roadmap: Report the target sedation score and ask: where is the patient going? Report the current level of sedation and delirium assessment (pain scoring can be incorporated) and ask: where is the patient now? Review the ongoing sedative, analgesia and antipsychotic requirements and ask: how did the patient get here?

Key points

- If you don't look for it, you will not find it.
- To monitor the patient's brain, first assess the sedation score then screen for delirium.
- Intubated critical care patients can be screened for delirium using either the CAM-ICU or the ICDSC – it is your choice.
- Implementing delirium screening needs education, persistence and more education.
- The value in screening resides in treating.

FURTHER READING

Training manual for CAM-ICU including frequently asked questions. www.icudelirium.org. Confusion Assessment Method: training manual freely available.

www.viha.ca/mhas/resources/delirium/tools.htm. This website has general delirium resources directed at the elderly including CAM training manual, relative information leaflets and posters.

http://www.learnicu.org/SiteCollectionDocuments/Pain,% 20Agitation,%20Delirium.pdf.

Brummel NE *et al*. Implementing delirium screening in the ICU: secrets to success. *Critical Care Medicine* 2013; 41(9): 2196–208.

Davis D and MacLullich A. Understanding barriers to delirium care: a multicentre survey of knowledge and attitudes amongst UK junior doctors. *Age and Ageing* 2009; 38: 559–63.

Chapter 8

How to prevent delirium?

Introduction

It is estimated that we can achieve a 30% risk reduction of delirium in a general hospital. In critical care we are often dealing with and treating consequences of illnesses or their complications. When it comes to delirium, however, we need to focus on prevention as the core strategy. The expression 'prevention is better than cure' is very much the case. Current prevention tactics are based on the risk factors outlined in Chapter 5.

Successfully preventing delirium

The few studies that have looked at the prevention of delirium have included elderly patients admitted following a fractured neck of femur, or other general medical conditions. These studies provide a disparate group of interventions. The landmark study done by Inouye *et al.* was published in the *New England Journal of Medicine* in 1999. In an elderly population (the average age was 80 ± 6 years), they attempted to address some of the problems from previous studies such as small samples, use of non-targeted

interventions and relatively insensitive outcome
measures. Moreover, they set out to compare matched
patients, with one receiving the interventions and one the
usual care.

When allocated to the intervention group, the patient was
entered into 'The Elder Life Program'. This addressed six
factors thought to be modifiable in clinical practice, using a
predefined protocol for each (Table 8.1).

Table 8.1 The six factors of the Hospital Elder Life
Program, and related actions for each factors

Cognitive impairment	The orientation protocol included the use of a white board with care-team member's names as well as establishing time and place with the patient 3 times a day
Sleep deprivation	The sleep-enhancement protocol used unit-wide noise reduction strategies such as vibrating bleepers as well as rescheduling medicine rounds to allow sleep time; as well as a non-pharmacological sleep protocol including a warm drink, relaxation tapes and a back massage
Immobility	The early mobilization protocol as well as active range of motion exercises included the minimal use of immobilizing equipment such as urinary catheters
Visual impairment Hearing impairment	Visual and hearing aids with adaptive equipment and daily reinforcement of their use addressed visual and hearing impairment
Dehydration	Dehydration was screened for and oral fluid intake encouraged in patients at risk

Reprinted with permission, THE HOSPITAL ELDER LIFE PROGRAM
(© 2000, SHARON K. INOUYE, MD, MPH).

Significantly, an implementation team worked in addition to the ward staff to enable the protocol implementation. This team included a geriatric nurse-specialist, two specially trained elder life specialists, a certified therapeutic-recreation specialist (sounds like a nice job!), a physiotherapist, a care of the elderly consultant and 40 volunteers. The volunteers were trained and each patient had 20 to 30 minutes three times a day of volunteer time.

Delirium developed in only 10% of patients in the intervention group, as opposed to 15% in the usual care group. The total number of days in delirium and the number of delirious episodes was much less in the intervention group. Receiving the intervention was also associated with less cognitive impairment on discharge and a significant reduction in the use of sleep medications.

The interventions were more successful in patients at intermediate risk of delirium than those at high risk. At the time Sharon Inouye remarked: 'Once delirium occurs, however, the cat's more or less out of the bag. The intervention has no significant effect on severity or recurrence, showing that prevention of delirium is much more effective than treatment.' The interventions used in this study represent a quality of care we would wish for all our elderly patients. In order to provide that care a whole additional team of professionals and volunteers was used. The balance between available resources and optimal clinical care can be challenging and may not allow us to formally implement this whole programme.

HELP: adhere to delirium prevention goals

A magic programme with additional resources used to implement a multi-component delirium prevention 'bundle' may be an answer, but how important is the attention to detail, adhering to each and every intervention? The increase in available resources may be the reason for success. Inouye decided to check this by evaluating whether the level of adherence had an impact on delirium. Results showed the risk of delirium was 89% lower in the highest adherence group when compared with the lowest adherence group. It was also shown that it was not one component that accounted for the effect, but several components had to be applied together for maximum effect.

Inouye and co-workers concluded that it was necessary to target all the six areas to achieve maximum benefit. They observed that compliance was important in both non-pharmacological and pharmacological interventions.

The Hospital Elder Life Program (HELP) continues today as an innovative strategy for elderly patients using tested delirium prevention interventions to improve quality of hospital care (see their website address at the end of this chapter).

Surprisingly, but in keeping with other similar observations, a 6-month telephone interview follow-up of the surviving patients did not show a maintained improvement in outcomes. The intervention appeared however still to have beneficial effects on self-rated health and functional status in the patients in the high-risk groups.

Delirium prevention programs put to the test

The effectiveness of an evidence-based ICU delirium prevention bundle called ABCDE and developed by Wes Ely and colleagues was subject to a quality improvement project in an 18-month before and after study. A flowchart based on sedation, delirium and mobilization was put into practice.

The implementation of the ABCDE bundle in a diverse group of critically ill patients decreased the number of patients with delirium from 49%, before ABCDE bundle care, to 62% following implementation. It also resulted in less time spent on mechanical ventilation.

In contrast, an enhanced exercise and cognitive programme of progressive resistance exercise, mobilization and orientation set outside of critical care was not effective in reducing the incidence of delirium when compared with usual care. Tested in 648 medical inpatients in Australia, it showed a lower incidence of delirium in the intervention group (4.9% vs. 5.9% for usual care) but had no effect on delirium duration or severity, or discharge destination or length of stay. A geriatric liaison intervention tested in the Netherlands to prevent post-operative delirium in 260 frail elderly cancer patients that

Table 8.2 ABCDE prevention bundle

A = Awakening, daily awakening trial

B = Breathing, spontaneous breathing trial

C = Co-ordination of awakening and breathing trials

D = Delirium monitoring/management

E = Early exercise mobility

included a geriatric consultation, treatment plan targeted at individual risk factors, daily visits and advice made no difference to the incidence of delirium (9.4% in intervention group vs. 14.3% in usual care group). Finally, a UK randomized controlled trial of 600 patients tested best practice care for patients with delirium or dementia against standard acute geriatric or medical ward care. While there was improved experience for patients and carers (not to be underestimated), the study showed no difference in the main outcome (time spent at home 90 days after randomization) and it was concluded that there were no convincing healthcare benefits.

These interventions are examples of excellent clinical practice and show that some outcomes cannot be quantified. The challenge is to justify the resources required to implement a quality intervention directed at delirium and related outcomes without clear evidence of benefit.

'Delirium care bundle'

In order to reduce delirium we need to look beyond the admission diagnosis and consider the whole physiological status of our patients as regards risk factors for delirium. . .

All our patients need the quality care that delirium prevention entails, e.g. a good night's sleep, attention to hydration and keeping them moving.

Clinical practice guidelines developed in the UK and in Australia agree that hospital-based multi-component preventative strategies have good enough evidence to support their use.

Target care to delirium

Specialized or targeted care will decrease delirium. The best example is shown in a study where elderly patients with a fracture of the neck of the femur had 35% to 65% risk of developing delirium. A structured geriatric consultation preoperatively or within 24 hours of surgery decreased the incidence of delirium by over one third, when compared to standard care. It also reduced severe delirium by over 50% with an overall number needed to treat of 5.6 (you only need to see 6 patients to help one of them!).

But what was done? Standard care meant management by the orthopaedic team and ad-hoc involvement of physicians on a reactive rather than proactive basis. A structured geriatric consultation consisted of ten modules, each consisting of two to five recommendations (Table 8.3). These recommendations were prioritized to improve adherence and limited to no more

Table 8.3 Modules to be checked while applying standard delirium care

Adequate oxygen delivery

Fluid/electrolyte balance

Treatment of severe pain

Elimination of unnecessary medications

Regulation of bowel/bladder function

Adequate nutritional intake

Early mobilization and rehabilitation

Prevention, early detection and treatment of major post-operative complications

Appropriate environmental stimuli

Treatment of agitated delirium

than five after the initial visit, and no more than three in the subsequent follow-up visits.

Patients who are cared for by informed staff familiar with delirium will benefit. Either they will not become delirious or suffer shorter episodes. This then translates into a reduction in length of stay and in some cases even reduced mortality.

A care of the elderly ward which routinely applies the principles of risk reduction or a specialized delirium ward where patients with prevalent delirium can be admitted for management are two examples of targeted care that have benefits. Both reduce either the incidence or duration of delirium. For those of us who work in hospitals without the imagination or resources to support such a facility, it is something to work towards.

In the meantime education is key in motivating staff to think about how they can reduce delirium in their patients.

Educate the staff

Delirium is poorly understood, particularly in ICU patients. It has been shown that trainee doctors lack the basic knowledge required to diagnose and manage delirium, rather than lacking awareness of its high prevalence and clinical significance. An educational package on delirium will decrease its prevalence in older medical inpatients. The teaching has to be directed at medical and nursing staff. It need not be lengthy or expensive but will require resources and time, from both trainers and trainees.

Directing the programme at a specific patient group or particular risk factors will be important, for example increasing the awareness of the role of steroids in delirium when teaching trainee anaesthetists in choosing which drugs to use for post-operative nausea and vomiting.

Implementing delirium screening in a unit must include an ongoing educational programme. Education is fundamental.

Reduce restraints – mobilize!

Early mobilization will decrease delirium and increase the number of patients who achieve activities of daily living on discharge (see Table 4.1 in Chapter 4). Physical restraints are recognized risk factors for delirium. These are not generally used in the UK but are in other countries. However, practitioners attach a number of unrecognized medical restraints such as urinary catheters, electrocardiogram leads or other lines.

Consider what restricts the patient's movements unnecessarily. Routine devices should be removed as soon as the patient's condition allows. This is particularly the case in patients who are waiting on an ICU for a ward bed to become available. How often will a patient become delirious while waiting, leading to an extended stay in the unit?

Early mobilization of patients is good for a number of reasons, including maintenance of muscle mass and power, reduction in thromboembolic events and chest infections. Early active and passive physiotherapy tailored to the patient's clinical state decreases the duration of delirium and subsequently the length of stay in ICU. Early mobilization requires good pain relief.

Kill the pain

Pain relief is important and the use of morphine or regional block is effective in modifying the incidence of delirium in elderly patients, from the patients with a fracture through to the ones in ICU with major burn injuries.

Avoiding opioids or administering very low doses when patients are in pain is associated with increased risk of delirium (apart from being poor clinical practice). Delirium can be an important and unrecognized factor associated with rapidly escalating pain – such as with progressive cancer. Patients with delirium may require a greater amount of breakthrough analgesia at night because of sleep–wake disturbance.

It is challenging balancing the risks of opioid drugs precipitating delirium in a patient against the risk and suffering caused by pain itself.

A 63-year-old man with lung cancer invading the chest wall with destruction of several ribs was treated with radiation therapy, oral morphine and non-steroidal analgesics. The pain associated with radiotherapy was relieved with increasing doses of morphine but there were still unpredictable episodes of severe pain. Within days,

*paroxysms of pain were accompanied by marked agitation.
The patient became irritable and inattentive but denied any
anxiety, depression or confusion; only complaining about the
severity and frequency of the painful episodes. After many days of
ineffective management with escalating doses of opioid, during which
the episodes of agitation, inattention and confusion increased, the
staff considered whether delirium was a contributing factor to his
distress. He was given haloperidol 1 mg twice a day orally. Within
1 day his requests for analgesics decreased and his mental status
improved.*

(Adapted from Coyle *et al.* [10].)

*A 59-year-old man with metastatic non-small-cell lung cancer was
admitted with progressive lower extremity weakness and instability.
Two years previously he had developed brain metastases following
which he had radiotherapy. He had decided on palliative comfort care
at home. Before admission, he became irritable and unco-operative
and a brain CT scan suggested increasing mass effect of the metastases.
When admitted in the emergency room, he was given lorazepam to
control his irritability and agitation. He became worse and fell while
trying to get out of bed. He was physically restrained and admitted to a
palliative care unit. In the palliative care suite the restraints were
removed and he was attended by a 24-hour sitter. His agitation was
believed to be due in part to uncontrolled pain and morphine was
titrated to control pain, following which his agitation was significantly
decreased although still a problem. Dexamethasone and lorazepam
were stopped and he was started on haloperidol. His partner brought
in his favourite music. These measures helped him to settle and he
was transferred to a residential hospice on fentanyl patch, haloperidol
and lorazepam as needed for insomnia or anxiety only. He died
4 days later.*

(Adapted from Breitbart and Alici [11].)

Control sedation

The way sedation is administered in an ICU can be as important as the type of sedative agents in use. Sedation protocols must include the routine use of sedation scoring, daily sedation targets and monitoring.

Clinicians should pay the same attention to the level of sedation as they give to the blood pressure. This means titrating drugs to a target aimed at ensuring the patient's pain relief and comfort while maintaining communication. This is a key message from the Pain, Agitation and Delirium management guidelines written by the American Critical Care Society. Various sedation score tools are available and each unit will have its own preference.

More than 23 sedation bedside assessments have been used in the ICU, only four of which were initially published as validated tools. The Richmond Agitation-Sedation Scale differentiates between response to verbal stimulus as opposed to a response to physical stimulus and is a good tool to monitor arousal, the first step to monitoring the brain (see Chapter 7). In the UK two thirds of units use the Ramsay scale which was described in 1974. Its popularity is likely attributable to its availability and ease of use.

Unless clinically indicated, sedated ventilated patients should be maintained at a level of responsiveness to verbal stimulus. The sedative drug should be stopped if the level of sedation is too deep, then restarted at a lower dose once the target is reached.

Some intensivists claim that benzodiazepines should not be used at all to sedate ICU patients. All psychoactive drugs have been implicated in the development of delirium, but the evidence implicating benzodiazepines is overwhelming, especially when compared with propofol. This has been challenged in a study in 99 patients that showed that while duration of coma is related to the use of benzodiazepines, delirium is not. The Canadian protocolized analgesia, sedation and delirium trial, which demonstrated a reduction in coma and delirium, and better analgesia, included the use of midazolam or propofol.

Ketamine, occasionally used as a last resort in the difficult-to-ventilate asthmatic, is known to cause post-operative hallucinations. Some may remember old 'K' signs, these were hung at the end of a patient's bed in the post-anaesthetic recovery area as a warning to staff not to disturb this patient unnecessarily – they had received ketamine! The popular anaesthetic volatile agent sevoflurane is now thought to cause post-operative agitation in children when used to maintain anaesthesia.

In summary, it is better to limit the total exposure of patients to any sedative drug while maintaining good analgesia. The intelligent use of agents tailored to a patient's responses will enable a patient to write notes while on full ventilation, opiate infusion (in our experience, fentanyl) and low-dose sedation.

Once we are using good sedation practices, monitoring our patients' brains, treating pain, relieving anxiety and enabling sleep, the incidence of delirium in our ventilated patients will decrease.

Two more newer drugs could potentially be very useful indeed: remifentanil and dexmedetomidine.

Remifentanil is an ultra short-acting opioid given by infusion that has been shown to decrease the time patients spend on ventilators and to reduce delirium in elective post-operative patients.

Dexmedetomidine is an alpha 2 receptor agonist used as a sedative in ICU and has been available in the USA since 1999 and Europe since 2011. It is a highly selective alpha 2 receptor agonist and acts in the locus coeruleus. It has a distribution phase of around 6 minutes and a half-life of 2 hours. ICU trials comparing dexmedetomidine infusion with benzodiazepines have shown a clinically significant reduction in the prevalence of delirium. Dexmedetomidine has also been shown to reduce post-operative delirium in cardiac surgical patients.

Dexmedetomidine is clinically effective, has opiate-sparing properties and is well tolerated. It is more effective in maintaining light sedation as compared with standard practice early in critical care stay. Arousability, communication, and patient co-operation are better with dexmedetomidine sedation than with midazolam and propofol (MIDEX/PRODEX study) although patient response can be variable. The vast majority of ICU patients will not need a bolus of dexmedetomidine as they usually have already received other sedating drugs. This decreases the risk of side effects such as bradycardia or hypotension, although these may sometimes be welcome in the ICU patient. The original studies used lower doses for up to 24 hours, but subsequent studies (MENDS and SEDCOM) have shown safety with doses up to 2 µg/kg/h for long duration, although with an increased incidence of side

effects (bradycardia and hypotension that resolve when
stopping the drug with no other intervention usually required).

Clonidine is another alpha 2 agonist that is regularly used by
many European intensivists, particularly in the context of
alcohol withdrawal. There are very limited trial data for
clonidine and the clinical use is based on experience.
Clonidine affinity for the alpha 2 receptors is much less than
dexmedetomidine but both agents have analgesic and sedative
properties. It can be administered enterally or as an infusion
and has similar effects to dexmedetomidine on blood pressure
and heart rate.

Using drugs to prevent delirium

There is not enough evidence currently to support the use of
prophylactic antipsychotics in order to prevent delirium in
critically ill patients.

The Hope-ICU trial, a randomized double-blind trial
comparing early intravenous haloperidol with placebo in
142 ventilated patients, did not show a decrease in delirium when
haloperidol was given early in the patient stay regardless of
whether patients were in coma or screened positive for delirium.

The main point regarding delirium prevention and drugs is
that many drugs are deliriogenic, in particular those with
anticholinergic properties or the GABA (γ-aminobutyric acid)
agonists. There is more information about drugs as risk factors
for delirium in Chapter 5. Critical care patients are exposed to
numerous medications, and the best prevention of delirium
remains in stopping any drug no longer required.

What about alcohol withdrawal?

Numerous guidelines exist on how to treat alcohol withdrawal (refer to the list of further reading at the end of this chapter). The patients who are at risk of delirium tremens are often given benzodiazepines (usually chlordiazepoxide) and vitamins (thiamine and vitamin C). Haloperidol is used to treat psychotic episodes. More is explained in Chapter 9, in the miscellaneous drugs section.

Key points

- Education of the clinical team is key in preventing delirium.
- Strategies to minimize risks should be defined and structured; and part of routine care.
- Strategies include orientation, communication, early mobilization and rationalizing drug exposure.
- Good analgesia and sedation protocols are needed – and will decrease the incidence of delirium.

FURTHER READING

Barr J, *et al*. Clinical practice guidelines for the management of pain, agitation, and delirium in adult patients in the intensive care unit. *Critical Care Medicine* 2013; 41: 263–306.

Lonergan E *et al*. Antipsychotics for delirium. *Cochrane Database of Systematic Reviews* 2007, Issue 2. Art No: CD005594.

Siddiqi N *et al.* Interventions for preventing delirium in hospitalised patients. *Cochrane Database of Systematic Reviews* 2007, Issue 2. Art No: CD005563.

Safer Healthcare Now – Canadian Initiative; Prevention and Management of Delirium. www.saferhealthcarenow.ca/EN/ Interventions/DeliriumPrevention/Documents/Delirium% 20Getting%20Started%20Kit.pdf.

The Hospital Elder Life Program (HELP). http://www. hospitalelderlifeprogram.org/public/public-main.php.

Chapter 9

Treatment of delirium in critical care

Introduction

Considering the seriousness of delirium, it is surprising (and frustrating) that the availability of effective pharmacological treatments is limited. This is explained in part by the fact that the pathophysiology is poorly understood – as outlined in Chapter 4. As a clinical syndrome, delirium can be compared to the acute respiratory distress syndrome (ARDS) that has similarly poor outcomes with no magic bullet to make it all better.

Do the drugs used for delirium rectify the neurotransmitter balance or simply alleviate the symptoms? Should we use drugs to treat delirium at all? Not according to the American Pain, Delirium and Analgesia guidelines, pointing out that there are insufficient data to recommend their use.

As with many conditions in ICU, the most important aspect of treatment is determining and dealing with the cause(s) of the problem. You cannot beat delirium if you do not address all treatable precipitating factors.

Identify and treat the cause

Delirium is always triggered by some 'event'. It may be a relatively small insult in the vulnerable patient, for instance a new urinary tract infection or a single dose of zopiclone in an elderly patient with pre-existing cognitive impairment. Keep in mind that the two commonest causes of new onset delirium in ICU are infection and drugs. Importantly, remember that simple measures such as restoring oxygenation and blood pressure may be enough to clear delirium in a sick patient. Delirium is an early clinical sign not to be ignored!

Screening for delirium is just a part of the whole war against it. A full medical history should be taken and any predisposing features for developing delirium noted. In particular it is important to establish whether the patient has had any cognitive impairment prior to admission, and if so, to what degree. If a patient is at high risk of developing delirium (e.g. has mild dementia), the search for a specific cause may be difficult. In a young usually fit patient the cause is often fairly obvious.

The patient should be examined and appropriate investigations undertaken; infective and metabolic causes should be sought. Remember that in many patients there may be more than one precipitating cause.

A notable case report describes an 85-year-old patient with cognitive impairment admitted to a specialized delirium ward in a Swedish hospital. Her final diagnoses turned out to be (1) acute myocardial infarction, (2) haemolytic anaemia, (3) diabetes mellitus, (4) urinary tract infection, (5) fresh fractures in the right hip and (6) constipation. Her delirium cleared after her somatic illnesses were treated.

A patient who was on a small dose of norepinephrine to maintain her mean arterial pressure but was otherwise doing well and starting to sit out of bed for short periods screened positive for delirium. On reviewing her drug chart she had been started on steroids the previous day for a 'soft' reason. These were stopped and by the following day her delirium had cleared.

A patient with an acute exacerbation of chronic obstructive airways disease was admitted with mixed delirium. Her delirium cleared with the use of non-invasive ventilation and normalization of her $PaCO_2$. She did however require one dose of intravenous haloperidol initially so she would tolerate the mask.

A patient became CAM-ICU positive 2 days after stopping haemofiltration for acute-on-chronic renal failure. The renal support was restarted and once his electrolytes were back to normal so was his mental status!

Delirious patient? Consult 'Dr DRE'

Before reaching for the prescription chart review, the clinician may want to consult Dr DRE (**D**iseases, **D**rug **R**emoval, **E**nvironment). Dr DRE will look for diseases (sepsis, congestive heart failure), attempt to remove drugs (stop deliriogenic medications) and try to modify the environment (orientate, aid sleep, mobilize).

Pharmacological treatment: haloperidol

Antipsychotic drugs are used because delirium involves an imbalance of neurotransmitters: a central cholinergic deficiency and a relative excess of dopamine occur in patients with delirium.

Theoretically D2 receptor blockade plus an associated enhanced acetylcholine release should restore the imbalance of neurotransmitters in the brain. It is, however, more complicated than that, as will be explained.

Antipsychotics are used in a range of severe psychiatric disorders including the short-term treatment of acute psychotic, manic and psychotic–depressive disorders as well as agitated dementia; and the long-term treatment of chronic psychotic disorders including schizophrenia. Antipsychotics

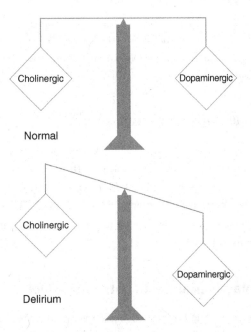

Figure 9.1 Delirium is the result of an imbalance between dopaminergic and cholinergic pathways.

are the mainstay of drug therapy when treating patients with delirium, and the most commonly used is haloperidol.

At the very least they can modify the symptoms of delirium.

A history of antipsychotics

The first antipsychotic used in the treatment of hallucinations and delusions in schizophrenia was chlorpromazine. The convoluted path that led to chlorpromazine started in 1856 with an exquisite purple dye. From this came methylene blue which Ehrlich observed was effective in treating the symptoms of malaria. This was resurrected during the twentieth-century world wars when some countries were cut off from the primary supplies of quinine and looked for a synthetic substitute. The phenothiazine derivative compounds were eventually found not to possess significant antimalarial properties, but were interesting because of their antihistamine effects. This work resulted in promethazine. In 1950, it was demonstrated that promethazine potentiated other anaesthetic agents and the search started for derivatives with similar activity. Chlorpromazine was tested in a 57-year-old labourer admitted to hospital for erratic uncontrollable behaviour; he had made impassioned political speeches in cafes, proclaimed a love of liberty while walking down the street with a flowerpot and intermittently assaulted strangers. Within a day on chlorpromazine he was calm and after 3 weeks appeared nearly normal. This and subsequent clinical successes with chlorpromazine stimulated the widespread

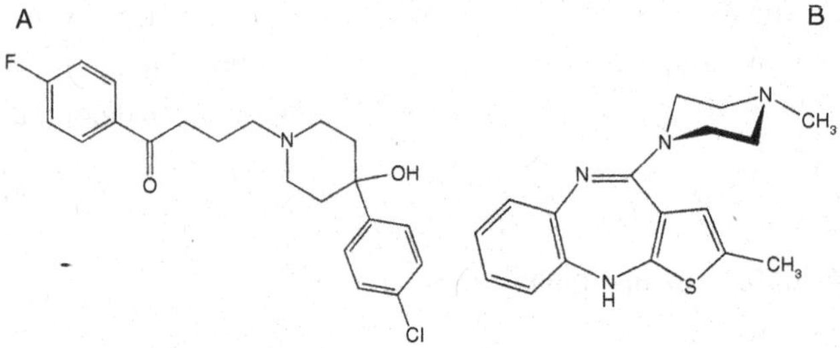

Figure 9.2 Chemical structure of haloperidol (A) and olanzapine (B).

search for other antipsychotic drugs. A Belgian physician, Dr Paul Janssen, was working on derivatives of pethidine to develop more potent opioid analgesics (and managed to develop fentanyl, alfentanil, sufentanil, droperidol and etomidate amongst others). The incorporation of a butyrophenone group led to a drug with notable cataleptic effects which reminded Janssen of chlorpromazine. Numerous derivatives were produced, one of which was haloperidol, so called because of the two halogenated substitutes incorporated into the molecule.

Mode of action of antipsychotics

Most typical antipsychotics block dopamine receptors in the mesolimbic system. The conventional antipsychotics – chlorpromazine and haloperidol – also block dopamine receptors in the nigrostriatal system (which results in extrapyramidal side effects) and in the tubero-infundibular pathway (explaining the effects on prolactin levels). Clozapine was introduced in 1966 and was effective against the positive symptoms of schizophrenia (hallucinations and delusions) but did not cause extrapyramidal side effects (and that is why it is called atypical). PET brain scans show that while typical neuroleptic antipsychotics block 80% to 90% of dopamine D2 receptors, clozapine only blocks 30% of D2 receptors with a greater occupancy of D1 receptors. Clozapine is also a potent blocker of 5-HT2 receptors.

Various antipsychotics act at different receptors with greater or lesser affinity, as shown in Figure 9.3. A list of antipsychotics, with some of their properties, is given in Table 9.1.

What is haloperidol?

Haloperidol is a butyrophenone first used clinically in 1957. It was hailed as a breakthrough in the treatment of schizophrenia and is said to be the greatest advance of twentieth-century psychiatry.

Haloperidol can be administered orally, subcutaneously, intramuscularly or intravenously. It is currently the only antipsychotic that can be administered intravenously and is usually administered as a slow bolus, although it has been given as an infusion. It is often used as a subcutaneous infusion in palliative care, usually combined in the same syringe as an opioid, sometimes with an antiemetic. It is extensively metabolized in the liver and its bioavailability when administered orally is around 60%.

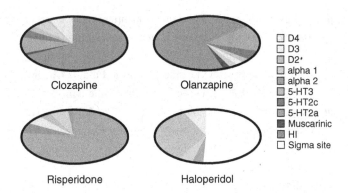

Figure 9.3 Receptor occupancy for various routinely used antipsychotics. It is likely that there is some variation from patient to patient. Adapted from Geri P *et al.* Conventional and atypical antipsychotics in the elderly: a review. *Clinical Drug Investigation* 2003; 23: 287–322. Adis Data Information BV.

Haloperidol's main action is as a dopamine antagonist in the central nervous system. It exhibits partial selectivity for D2 receptors particularly in the corpus striatum, thought to be responsible for its antipsychotic properties. It also acts on some alpha adrenoreceptors (α–1), opioid, muscarinic cholinergic, histaminergic and serotoninergic receptors.

Studies in newly diagnosed schizophrenic patients demonstrated that the D2 receptors have to be occupied at 65% for a clinical effect to be seen. Motor symptoms become apparent at 78% occupancy. However, there is a wide variation in measured D2 occupancy between patients taking the same dose of haloperidol. It is important to note that the findings of studies on patients with schizophrenia may not necessarily apply to critically ill patients with delirium.

Table 9.1 Neuroleptics that may be useful in managing delirium in elderly cancer patients.

Medication	Approximate daily dosage range	Available routes	Comments
Typical neuroleptics			
Haloperidol	0.5 to 5 mg every 2 to 12 h	Oral; intravenous; intramuscular	Watch for extrapyramidal symptoms
Chlorpromazine	12.5 to 50 mg every 4 to 12 h	Oral; intravenous; intramuscular	Watch for anticholinergic and cardiovascular effects; very sedating; orthostatic hypotension
Atypical neuroleptics			
Risperidone	0.25 to 2 mg every 12 h	Oral; depot intramuscular; orally dispersible tablets	Mildly sedating
Olanzapine	2.5 to 5 mg every 12 h	Oral; intramuscular; orally dispersible tablets	Sedating
Quetiapine	25 to 100 mg every 12 h	Oral	Most sedating
Ziprasidone	20 to 60 mg every 12 h	Oral; intramuscular	Less sedating
Aripiprazole	2.5 to 10 mg every 12 h	Oral	Less sedating

Reprinted with permission from Winell J and Roth AJ. Psychiatric assessment and symptom management in elderly cancer patients. *Oncology (Williston Park)* 2005; 19(11): 1479–90. UBM Medica. All rights reserved.

Table 9.2 Haloperidol pharmacodynamic properties

Half-life	12–35 hours (average 16 h)
Oral availability	44–75% (> 60%)
Volume of distribution	1280–2130 L
Time to steady state	7–10 days
Protein binding	91.5%
Time to peak plasma concentration	intravenous – 5–15 minutes oral – 4 to 6 h
Decay post peak	intravenous – steep over 1 h then exponential oral – slow exponential

Vella-Brincat J and Macleod AD. Haloperidol in palliative care. *Palliative Medicine* 18(3): 195–201, Copyright © 2004 Sage Publications. Reprinted by permission of SAGE.

Why use haloperidol?

For years the evidence regarding the use of haloperidol to treat delirium was based on case series and case reports. Haloperidol has been used in tens of thousands of patients throughout the world for years.

The majority of patients (no less than 72% quoted) who remember the experience of being delirious found it distressing, regardless of whether it was hypoactive or hyperactive. Some patients still maintain the fixed belief that members of ICU staff were trying to kill them or remove their organs, even though they know and accept that they were delirious. Clinicians may use haloperidol in delirious patients simply with the aim of reducing these frightening perceptual disturbances.

Haloperidol is the traditional first-line drug recommended to treat delirium in any national or international guidelines that recommend a drug treatment. The available evidence for the management of delirium is limited and guidelines reflect this, for instance the dose of haloperidol varies tenfold. The 2013 US Pain, Delirium and Analgesia guidelines published by the American College of Critical Care Medicine in conjunction with the Society of Critical Care Medicine and American Society of Health-System Pharmacists concluded there was no published evidence that haloperidol reduces the duration of delirum. A phase 2 trial of 141 ventilated patients comparing haloperidol with placebo supported this by showing no difference in the duration of delirium between treated and non-treated patients, even though the study reported a decrease in agitation with improvement over the study period in patients who received haloperidol.

The UK National Institute for Health and Care Excellence (NICE) guidelines are not specific to critical care patients. They recommended that the use of antipsychotics be limited to use in patients who are agitated when a danger to themselves or staff. In a UK survey of intensive care consultants, 74% use haloperidol as first-line treatment for hyperactive delirium and of those who treat hypoactive delirium pharmacologically, 80% use haloperidol. As delirium has become more frequently recognized in our critically ill patients the use of haloperidol has become more widespread, but this may have been tempered by the results of this UK phase 2 trial.

What dose?

The initial dose of haloperidol recommended in the British National Formulary by intramuscular or intravenous injection is 2 to 10 mg (note that haloperidol is not approved for intravenous use in the USA).

Critically ill patients with hyperactive delirium are often a danger to themselves and to staff. They are usually connected to a number of support devices. They are at risk of accidental extubation, disconnection of arterial lines and loss of intravenous cannulae. Rapid control is needed and intensivists will use higher doses than used elsewhere in the hospital. Indeed in the past haloperidol has been given in very high doses with minimal side effects. There are reports of doses up to 975 mg! (not a typo error, but nine hundred and seventy-five mg) having been given to individual patients within 24 hours, on occasion as a continuous infusion.

Current ICU clinical practice is to use an initial dose of 2.5 to 5 mg haloperidol intravenously, and then add more and maybe more, and sometimes even more, and why not even some more, as required. In general, less haloperidol is being given per dose although more patients are receiving it. This trend will probably continue. The lower dose is used in elderly patients. Outside of the ICU, lower doses are used in elderly patients. In these cases, the clinicians prescribe enteral haloperidol, which is associated with more extrapyramidal side effects, and they are looking for an improvement over days to weeks. As intravenous haloperidol can take up to 30 minutes to act, some older, less often used regimens are based on incremental administration at 30- to 60-minute intervals, others 6 to 12 hourly.

Doses of haloperidol used in delirium are variable and it is difficult to suggest a range that all clinicians who come across delirium (virtually all clinicians!) will agree to use. Personally, the authors of this book aim to use the minimum dose required for the shortest time possible, and only after non-pharmacological interventions and cessation of potentially precipitating drugs have failed. Screening regularly for delirium (at least once per shift or when needed) is important to ensure we use only what is required.

Haloperidol should be avoided in patients following traumatic brain injury. The main mechanism of traumatic brain injury in high-speed collision is diffuse axonal injury. Diffuse axonal injury is associated with a reduction in dopamine turnover so giving these patients a potent dopamine antagonist may aggravate the brain injury. In these patients, olanzapine is the drug of choice (but this assertion is based on only two case reports).

Risks of haloperidol

Haloperidol is generally considered to be a safe drug, in and outside of critical care. An advantage is the absence of respiratory depression and limited haemodynamic effects.

Before using haloperidol, obtain a 12-lead electrocardiogram and record the duration of the QTc interval; measure the electrolytes and correct the potassium and magnesium levels whenever required. Torsades de pointes has been reported with the use of haloperidol as a relatively rare but dangerous side effect. Most clinicians will restrict haloperidol's use when the patient's QTc is over 500 msec. This is a life-threatening multiform ventricular arrhythmia that frequently degenerates into ventricular fibrillation. Torsades de pointes usually develops (but not always) after large doses of haloperidol and typically in patients with prolonged QTc intervals. Torsades de pointes has also been associated with hypokalaemia, hypocalcaemia, hypomagnesaemia and hypothyroidism. Treatment includes magnesium (one of the few good reasons to give magnesium) and cardioversion as required.

The parenteral administration of haloperidol causes fewer extrapyramidal side effects than when given enterally. Extrapyramidal side effects include twitching around the mouth and a fine tremor in the hands that are reversible unless the drug is continued for several weeks. They are treated by reducing or stopping haloperidol. If symptomatic treatment is needed for acute dystonia, procyclidine 5 to 10 mg or diphenhydramine 50 mg can be given intravenously.

Akathisia is a restlessness that may be confused with agitation. If severe it can be extremely distressing to the patient, who feels the need to move constantly. It can be assessed by both observing the patient and asking them directly – assuming they are able to communicate.

Neuroleptic malignant syndrome is a rare and serious side effect of haloperidol with a mortality of around 10%. It is an idiosyncratic reaction to the drug characterized by fever,

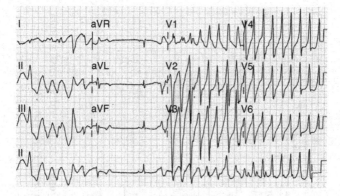

Figure 9.4 Torsades de pointes induced by haloperidol. Reprinted with permission from Prof. Jirina Martinkova, and Prof. Jiri Kvasnicka, Long-QT-interval syndrome, polymorphic ventricular tachycardia (torsade de pointes). www./fhk.cuni.cz/farmakol/anglicka/hughes/html/QTinterval/QThistory.htm.

severe muscle rigidity and autonomic changes such as a labile blood pressure. It is a diagnosis of exclusion and many of the features such as high temperature, metabolic acidosis and elevated creatine kinase can be seen for other reasons in critically ill patients. It is associated with the use of antipsychotics and 66% of cases present within a week of starting the drug. The incidence in all antipsychotic use is probably less than 0.1% although higher incidences have been documented. The reported incidence has decreased in the general psychiatric population probably because of lower doses of antipsychotics and the greater use of atypical antipsychotics. Treatment is supportive and intravenous dantrolene is used if the muscle rigidity is severe – 1 to 2.5 mg/kg initially then

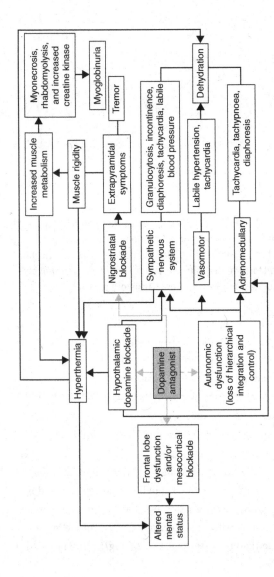

Figure 9.5 Proposed mechanism for the neuroleptic malignant syndrome. Adapted with permission from Strawn J. Neuroleptic malignant syndrome. *American Journal of Psychiatry* 2007; 164: 870–6.

1 mg/kg 6 hourly if improvement is seen with the first dose. Neuroleptic malignant syndrome is self-limiting once the drug is stopped. Interestingly, if the patients need antipsychotics (such as in cases of schizophrenia), 87% will be able to tolerate another antipsychotic later despite an episode of neuroleptic malignant syndrome.

Haloperidol, good or bad?

Enthusiastic users of haloperidol in ICU refer to a retrospective cohort analysis on 989 patients ventilated for more than 48 hours, comparing the hospital mortality between patients who had received haloperidol within 48 hours of admission and those who had never received haloperidol, as shown in Figure 9.6. A study by Wang *et al.* showed a reduction in the incidence of post-operative delirium in elderly ICU patients who received less than 2 mg haloperidol as an infusion (23.2% in the control group compared to 15.3% of patients). This patient population was in a less sick group than generally seen in critical care and had an average Acute Physiology and Chronic Health Evaluation (APACHE) score lower than 9. In a quality improvement study, non-randomized and using historical controls, the administration of 1 mg/kg haloperidol 8 hourly to patients at high risk of developing delirium decreased the incidence of delirium and increased the number of delirum-free days.

Sceptics believe that it is unlikely that targeting neurotransmitters downstream of the powerful drivers of ICU delirium is an effective strategy given what we know about the

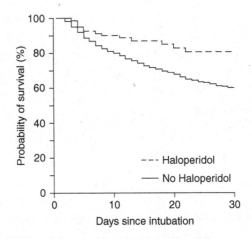

Figure 9.6 **Hospital mortality compared between patients who had haloperidol and those who did not. Reprinted with permission from Milbrandt E** *et al.* **Haloperidol use is associated with lower hospital mortality in mechanically ventilated patients.** *Critical Care Medicine* **2005; 33: 226–9.**

ongoing neuroinflammation and oxidative stress. In a double-blind, randomized, placebo-controlled trial in 141 ventilated patients, there was no difference seen in the duration of delirium or coma in patients who received a daily total dose of 7.5 mg.

Critics of the use of haloperidol point out adverse effects, in particular the prolongation of QT interval and the risk of inducing torsades de pointes.

Finally, there is no evidence to date that treating delirium improves patients' outcomes because the research has not been undertaken.

Other agents

Atypical antipsychotics

Atypical antipsychotics might be effective and safe in treating delirium but the evidence is limited. Atypical antipsychotics are the treatment of choice in patients where there are specific concerns about extrapyramidal symptoms.

Clozapine was described in 1988 and referred to as atypical because of the low risk of adverse extrapyramidal side effects. The term atypical has since been used for antipsychotic drugs manufactured from the 1990s, and includes drugs with variable neuro-pharmacodynamics. Atypical drugs bind more loosely to the D2 receptors than haloperidol, dissociate more rapidly and demonstrate a high level of serotonin receptor occupancy. The risk of extrapyramidal symptoms is usually lower.

There have been a handful of small case-controlled studies in the use of antipsychotic drugs for delirium. The three most studied agents are olanzapine, risperidone and quetiapine, they all have different affinities for dopamine and serotonin receptors (see Figure 9.3).

Olanzapine can be given intramuscularly or orally, at doses ranging from 5 to 10 mg. When initiating the treatment, higher doses are sometimes required, and to administer 10 mg several times over the first 24 hours is not uncommon and allows rapid control of symptoms. It is a useful alternative to haloperidol and can be used in combination in the acutely agitated delirious patient. When compared with haloperidol in critically ill patients, it has been shown to be as effective in treating delirium.

Quetiapine, when used in addition to haloperidol given by the bedside clinician to manage delirium, was shown in a small trial of 36 patients to result in faster resolution of delirium, less agitation, and faster transfer home or to rehabilitation.

In patients with traumatic brain injury where there are concerns over a relative dopamine deficiency, olanzapine is the preferred antipsychotic because of weaker D2 antagonistic properties as compared with haloperidol. Olanzapine can induce hyperlipidaemia and hyperglycaemia probably secondary to the blockade of neurotransmitters involved in glucose metabolism.

Like other atypical antipsychotics, risperidone has been shown to be as effective as haloperidol in the management of delirium but as with olanzapine there has been no placebo trial with sufficient numbers of patients to recommend these drugs routinely. A number of ICU clinicians regularly use these drugs for delirious patients, and claim to have good results. If a patient has mixed or agitated delirium which is not improving with haloperidol, it is certainly worth considering a short course of either of these drugs. Both drugs can only be given enterally.

Alpha 2 agonists

Dexmedetomidine is a highly selective alpha 2 agonist (see Chapter 8). Among four studies comparing dexmedetomidine and benzodiazepine strategies, three found that patients on dexmedetomidine were less likely to remain in delirium at the end of therapy, with reductions of 10% to 20% per day in delirium prevalence with dexmedetomidine.The US Pain, Analgesia and Delirium guidelines suggest that dexmedetomidine infusions be administered in preference to benzodiazepine infusions for sedation when a patient screens positive for delirium.

An open-label pilot study comparing dexmedetomidine with haloperidol for agitated intubated patients concluded that it was a promising agent. There are case reports regarding the successful use of dexmedetomidine in agitated patients with withdrawal syndromes and undergoing non-invasive ventilation. Conversely, a retrospective assessment of 40 patients hinted that transitioning to dexmedetomidine may be associated with increased agitation and pain, but this may have been due to improper dosage of other drugs.

Agitated delirium is a major challenge in critical care and dexmedetomidine is the obvious drug to research in these patients. While dexmedetomidine is expensive, a generic form may soon be available and likely to be cheaper. There is published evidence that costs of the drug as compared with midazolam are offset by days spent on mechanical ventilation, although these data were obtained in the context of an ongoing clinical efficacy trial with very strict criteria (SEDCOM).

Clonidine is a centrally acting antihypertensive drug, acting on alpha 2 adrenoreceptors. It has been used for years in anaesthetic practice mainly for its analgesic properties but more recently to prevent agitation associated with newer volatile anaesthetic agents. It can be used as a component of a multimodal sedation such as in patients who 'fight' the ventilator. It has sedative properties. There are a number of case reports of the use of clonidine in delirium tremens but the evidence is insufficient for it to be included in any guideline either in the UK or the USA. In the intubated patient, the addition of clonidine enterally or slowly intravenously 8 hourly can be very effective when a patient is requiring large doses of sedatives. An initial dose is 1 mcg/kg either enterally or diluted in saline and given over 10 to 15 minutes. At the very least it will decrease the amount of sedation required. A final word of caution is necessary as a few case reports have associated delirium with the use of clonidine.

Miscellaneous drugs

When faced with a delirious uncontrollable patient, anaesthetic drugs such as propofol are often used in small boluses. This is a short-term solution, and clinicians should remember that titrating propofol against its respiratory depressant and anaesthetic effects is difficult in the non-intubated patient. In the intubated patient, a propofol infusion is a means of controlling agitation. It is however not a replacement for analgesics if pain is suspected.

Benzodiazepines and delirium

Intravenous benzodiazepines are often used in combination with haloperidol when managing a hyperactive delirious patient, but benzodiazepines may precipitate and maintain a delirious state and are therefore not recommended.

It is sometimes the quickest and safest option for the agitated patient, and available to the staff in charge (but protocols could be developed in a unit to avoid this). Benzodiazepines will cause sedation and it might be required to institute or continue respiratory support.

An exception to this recommendation of avoiding benzodiazepines is in patients who are undergoing alcohol withdrawal. A meta-analysis demonstrated that giving benzodiazepines reduces the symptoms, duration and intensity of alcohol withdrawal. Benzodiazepines in this specific condition are associated with a risk reduction of seizures (7.7 per 100 patients treated). Chlordiazepoxide is commonly used in the UK, intravenous diazepam in the USA. All these patients need to be given thiamine to prevent serious neurological disorder and Wernicke's encephalopathy. Delirium developing in an alcoholic patient on benzodiazepines should be treated by adding in haloperidol, as described previously.

Acetylcholinesterase inhibitors

The association between delirium and a central cholinergic deficit led clinicians to think that anticholinesterase inhibitors, such as donepezil and rivastigmine, would be useful in the prevention and treatment of delirium.

A randomized controlled study in the Netherlands was terminated early for safety reasons after 104 of a planned 440 patients were recruited. Twelve patients who received rivastigmine as opposed to four in the placebo group died and the delirium was more severe and longer in patients receiving the drug.

The conclusion was clear – 'Rivastigmine does not decrease the duration of delirium and may increase mortality in critically ill patients'.

Sodium valproate

Intravenous valproic acid is a safe and effective anticonvulsant which acts by increasing the availability of γ-aminobutyric acid (GABA). There are several case reports about its use in psychiatric patients for the treatment of bipolar disorders and other aggressive or agitated states. Bourgeois *et al.* described six cases of patients with agitated delirium who had failed to respond with conventional therapy and then improved with the addition of sodium valproate.

Ondansetron

Ondansetron is worthy of a mention following a report from Turkey commenting on an open series of cardiac surgical patients. Thirty-four of thirty-five patients who developed symptoms of hyperactive delirium post-cardiac surgery showed a significant improvement following 8 mg of ondansetron intravenously. The theory is the antagonistic effects of ondansetron on the serotonin system. Again the evidence is too flimsy to recommend it and there is evidence that pure serotonin blockers are ineffective in delirium.

Adverse effects of treatment

In 2005, the US Food and Drug Administration issued a black box warning against the use of atypical antipsychotics in patients with dementia.

Research evaluating the association between the use of typical and atypical antipsychotics, adverse events and mortality has been published. The findings have been mixed because of differences in data source, methodological approach, sample size and geographical variation in treatment practices. Although some have detected an association between antipsychotic use and mortality, other studies report that antipsychotics have no effect – or even a protective effect – on mortality. All these studies probably fail to adequately control for confounding factors.

A study of 254 very frail, elderly demented patients concluded that neither the use of atypical antipsychotics nor conventional neuroleptics increased the hospital mortality or hospital admissions. The use of restraints, however, doubled the risk of mortality.

Similarly, the retrospective evaluation of the Medicare records of 2363 patients who resided in long-term care facilities found no evidence of increased hospital events or mortality when antipsychotics were used. These researchers took the functional status of the patients into account.

Drug treatment: what's missing?

To paraphrase Campbell *et al.*, we can say that the current literature lacks well-designed studies comparing interventions in a controlled environment. Future studies should include appropriate randomization and blinding techniques with adequate sample sizes in patient populations most likely to benefit to ensure accurate and reproducible outcome measurement.

Psychiatrists and delirium

Should we, or should we not, call the psychiatrist? Can we replace them with a screening tool, and then use haloperidol freely? Psychiatrists and intensivists may have different opinions on the matter, but we would advocate that a psychiatrist should be consulted for patients already under the care of a psychiatrist or on antipsychotic medications.

A psychiatrist is often helpful for patients whose agitation cannot be controlled with the usual measures, for patients with dementia when the diagnosis of delirium is proving uncertain, and in patients with persistent delirium.

Psychiatrists might be useful at a later stage, when patients are followed up and ICU-related post-traumatic stress disorder suspected.

Recipe ...

Identify and treat all possible causes.

If the QTc interval is greater than 450 msec, be careful. Do not use haloperidol at all if QTc greater than 500 msec.

If the QTc increases more than 25% from baseline, or increases to a value greater than 500 msec, stop antipsychotics.

Hyperactive delirium

Give haloperidol intravenously, choosing from 1 to 5 mg, according to patient age and weight.

Wait 30 minutes; if patient's agitation still not controlled double dose and repeat.

Wait 30 minutes; if patient's agitation still not controlled consider either double dose again and repeat or give olanzapine (intramuscularly or through a nasogastric tube).

If at any time the safety of the patient or the staff is compromised, use small boluses of fentanyl or propofol intravenously, and repeat as necessary (but be mindful of airway control).

Avoid the use of benzodiazepines except in patients with alcohol withdrawal.

Hypoactive delirium

Treating hypoactive delirium is based on non-pharmacological actions. Dr DRE (Diseases, Drug Removal, Environment) should be invited and the clinician will keep looking for and treating any reversible causes.

All non-pharmacological delirium interventions should be in place; in particular the patient should be mobilized.

Family and friends should be spoken to, so they and the patient can be reassured and motivated even if the prognosis is worse than for hyperactive delirium.

Key points

- Always seek and treat all possible causes of delirium.
- Haloperidol is the drug of choice for agitated delirium.
- Olanzapine is a parenteral alternative in the patient with prolonged QTc, or if suffering from Parkinson's disease, or when haloperidol does not work.
- Benzodiazepines should probably be avoided, except in patients withdrawing from alcohol where it must be given.

FURTHER READING

http://www.jwatch.org/fw107817/2013/08/22/follow-interview-delirium-and-intensive-care.

Dr DRE and Brain Road Map. www.icudelirium.org/docs/Implementation_Delirium_Screening.pdf.

Safer Healthcare Now – Canadian Initiative; Prevention and Management of Delirium. www.saferhealthcarenow.ca/EN/

Interventions/DeliriumPrevention/Documents/Delirium%
20Getting%20Started%20Kit.pdf.

Shen W. A history of antipsychotic drug development.
Comprehensive Psychiatry 1999; 40: 407–14.

Vella-Brincat J and Macleod AD. Haloperidol in palliative care.
Palliative Medicine 2004; 18: 195–201.

Chapter 10

Mental capacity and restraints

Catherine, 29, daughter of a doctor, suffered from severe asthma. She knew her illness well and while her attacks came on quickly she rapidly recovered and had never required intensive care. One Sunday morning she had a severe attack, her sister persuaded her to go to hospital on the understanding she would only be given oxygen. At the hospital she was given oxygen and a nebulizer which she said gave her a headache and she decided to leave the hospital. The clinical team looking after her were horrified having decided she needed intubation and ventilation from blood gas results. The emergency doctor contacted Catherine's father who asked her to wait until he arrived. In the meantime Catherine's condition improved and she tried to leave the hospital with her sister. She was taken back to her room, placed in four-point restraints and after 45 minutes was anaesthetized and intubated. The clinical team said later that after she was prevented from leaving she became more confused and combative, refusing treatment. She made a rapid recovery and was discharged the next day. Following this she had nightmares, cried constantly, was unable to return to work for several months and swore never to go back to hospital. Two years later she had another severe attack and became unconscious. Her brother called an ambulance and she was taken to a nearby hospital where she died after unsuccessful medical treatment.

(Adapted from Annas [12].)

Mental capacity

The US Supreme Court considered that there was no justification for the use of restraints in Catherine's care. Catherine did not lack capacity: she was able to make informed decisions about medical intervention. Physicians are required by law and ethics to obtain informed consent of patients before starting treatment. The UK and all 50 States of the USA have legislation that delineates the required standards for informed consent. In most countries any competent patient has the legal right to refuse medical intervention, for any reason, including no reason at all, even if that refusal appears absurd or harmful from the doctor's point of view.

It has been shown that more than three quarters of critically ill patients are unable to provide informed consent throughout an ICU stay, even after extubation. Patients with delirium lack the capacity to consent and are often subject to either physical or chemical restraint. Each country will have specific laws or guidance to protect individuals who are unable to make decisions for themselves which clinicians must be familiar with. For example in the UK, the Mental Capacity Act regulates what can or cannot be done.

In practice, it is down to the bedside clinician to decide whether a patient has capacity to understand, retain and process the given information and make an informed decision (rational or not). Assessment of capacity can be fraught with difficulty in patients with cognitive impairment or who are acutely ill.

To have capacity to consent to an intervention, a patient must be able to understand its nature, purpose and consequences, including possible adverse effects and the consequences of refusal. They need to be able to retain the information and be able to consider it long enough to be able to make a decision and then communicate this decision. This is key in how a clinician can ascertain capacity. In the case of Catherine the Supreme Court was quite clear, she knew what the physician wanted to do and why and she knew she could die if the intervention was not performed.

In delirious patients capacity assessment is complicated by the fluctuations in the level of consciousness and cognitive function.

Deprivation of liberty

Deprivation of liberty is a fundamental breach of human rights. In the USA, the fifth amendment clearly states that 'No person shall be . . . deprived of life, liberty or property, without due process of law'. In the UK, until the introduction of the Mental Capacity Act, there was no legal requirement to call individuals or organizations to account. This situation was corrected with the implementation of the Deprivation Of Liberty Safeguards, sometimes referred to as DOLS, which came out of the Mental Capacity Act. These apply to patients who lack capacity. In order for DOLS to apply, firstly a patient has to lack capacity, and secondly needs protection from harm in a way that may be seen as a deprivation of freedom, e.g. making them stay in bed.

Where does this leave the clinician?

Clinicians must be able to assess capacity. Lack of capacity in the sedated and ventilated patient is self-evident regardless of the presence or absence of delirium. Clinicians then base decisions on management as to what in the clinician's judgement is in the patient's best interests. In the situation of a patient who is obtunded with hypoxia and hypotension the immediate clinical need will dictate treatment unless there is a clear advance directive not to do so. In the patient who lacks capacity temporarily, such as one with delirium, efforts should be made to help the patient regain capacity so they can make decisions themselves. If the decision can wait until the patient regains capacity, then clinicians should wait.

A clinician should always document if a patient does not have capacity (and how the clinician came to this conclusion). In the ICU, other professionals are often involved in making this decision and they should document and corroborate the observations made. Local specialists in psychiatry (if available) should be able to help or advise.

In the vulnerable adult who does not have capacity, the clinicians should abide by local rules and laws. In the UK, the clinician needs to decide if Deprivation of Liberty standards apply – if they do apply, then the process prescribed by law must be adhered to (these go beyond the content of this book, but see the selected references at the end of the chapter). Health organizations must have systems in place to meet national legal requirements, protect vulnerable adults and advise clinicians when required.

An 83-year-old woman was admitted to hospital after hitting her head in a fall. A CT scan was negative; however, she was confused and disorientated. She asked to go home immediately. A psychiatric consultant decided she lacked capacity and she was kept in hospital for further evaluation.

A 72-year-old man with carcinoma of the colon refused preoperative testing. A consultant found him anxious, paranoid and psychotic, and treated him with olanzapine. The paranoid symptoms subsided, and he carried on with the tests.

A 52-year-old Spanish male with end-stage renal disease was admitted after a myocardial infarction. He refused dialysis and cardiac catheterization. With the insistence of an interpreter the psychiatrist determined he had capacity but was very frightened. With support from his family and an anxiolytic his anxiety diminished and he accepted the treatment recommendations.

A proportion of critically ill patients will go on to suffer persistent delirium, and the non-acute management of psychotic symptoms will be required after discharge from critical care. This may require applying for a Deprivation of Liberty authorization.

To restrain or not

Discussions regarding ethics, the law and delirium inevitably bring the issue of the use of restraints, whether physical or chemical. The use of physical restraints in intensive care varies enormously from place to place. Physical restraints are commonly used in some countries such as the USA, but are the exception in others such as the UK. In countries that don't use physical restraints, chemical restraints are used and thought to be, rightly or wrongly, more acceptable.

There is a justifiable groundswell of concern regarding the use of antipsychotics in patients with dementia for the purposes of 'crowd control' rather than in the patient's best interests. A number of warnings have been issued regarding what is perceived as the excessive use of antipsychotics in nursing homes and an apparent association with increased mortality.

Regarding deprivation of liberty, if it is established that a patient lacks capacity secondary to delirium, and needs to be restrained in order to treat a medically identified condition (e.g. to ensure that a patient does not remove life-supporting equipment such as an endotracheal tube), then restraints, chemical or physical, can be and should be used. In the UK, clinicians do not need to apply for a Deprivation of Liberty authorization in these circumstances. In the USA, a physician's order is required before restraints are used. In the USA, Federal Medicare regulations and policies, as well as the Joint Commission on the Accreditation of Healthcare Organizations (JCAHO), impose restrictions on the use of physical and chemical restraints. Most states also have laws governing the use of restraints – in a nutshell, they all demand that the least restrictive measure should be used for the shortest possible time, and the condition of the restrained patient must be continually assessed, monitored and re-evaluated. The same principles of minimal restraints for the shortest possible duration are also embedded in the UK Mental Capacity Act.

Physical restraints

With more publications reporting the risks of sedatives and prolonged ventilation, some clinicians are introducing the use of physical restraints to their units. The rationale is that more sedation will prolong the duration of ventilation and associated complications. Some clinicians consider that restraints such as mittens to stop the patient getting a grip on tubes are justified to decrease the risk of an increased amount of drugs and duration of ventilation.

There is however no evidence that the use of physical restraints decreases the risk of self-extubation or reduces length of stay. In contrast, physical restraints are a known risk factor for delirium. It is our belief that physical restraints should be used rarely, if ever, in the extremely elderly because of the risk of persistent delirium. Use of physical restraints for more than a day will impact on the mobility of the patients and this may hinder clinical recovery and be distressing. Always consider that patients may be trying to extubate themselves because they are ready to be extubated.

Soft wrist restraints that allow some arm movement may be helpful in selected delirious patients who absent-mindedly and repeatedly remove nasogastric tubes needed for enteral nutrition and medication.

The use of physical restraints on an ICU demands an organizational protocol to which all relevant healthcare clinicians – the multidisciplinary team – should be consulted on and have agreed upon. The protocol should be reviewed

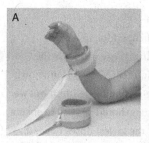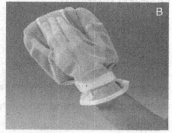

Figure 10.1 Example of physical restraints used to prevent the patient reaching for lines or tubes. A. Limb restraints. B. Posey glove.

by the Ethical Review Group in the organization. The protocol should include the circumstances in which restraints are used, the type of restraints, the frequency of review of the need for restraints (at least every 24 hours!) and the monitoring required. The protocol should make clear that clinicians should always document the reason for using or asking for restraints. It is an emotive subject and relatives, and hospital staff, may see restraints as distressing and undignified. The reasons for their use should be carefully explained to relatives and visitors. Reassurance should be given that they will be removed as soon as possible. The physician needs to discuss the need for restraint in each case with other healthcare professionals, especially the bedside nurses. Drugs or physical restraints should not be used as a means of convenience where convenience refers to an action to control or manage behaviour rather than treating the patient.

Chemical restraints

The use of antipsychotics, usually haloperidol, to control agitation is a chemical restraint: a drug is used to settle the patient down. As described in previous chapters, it is unknown whether antipsychotics are effective at treating delirium but we do know they decrease agitation. Drugs should be used to ensure patient and staff safety, and used at the lowest doses needed. Administering an antipsychotic drug to a terrified patient with or without additional sedation may modify their perceptual disturbances as well as control the agitation. Benzodiazepines are deliriogenic and should be reserved for management of a patient with extreme agitation. A Cochrane review from 2009 concluded that they are not indicated to manage hyperactive delirium because they can make the delirium worse. Quetiapine is a useful alternative to haloperidol if the patient can take tablets,

The hyperactive agitated delirious patient will inevitably be experiencing – and may later recall – frightening hallucinations, often believing their life or the lives of loved ones are at risk. Treatment should be our priority.

An ICU patient recalls: 'I had a mad, bad and most certainly psychotic 3 weeks in an ITU bed – intubated and delirious. I was absolutely sure [still am] that an ICU nurse tried to kill me to sell my organs on Ebay – heard the whole conversation whilst he was sedating me with serious drugs as I kept ripping out my central and trach ... I am OK now.'

The use of antipsychotics and physical restraints for persistent agitation symptoms is a reason to think of a patient as vulnerable, and assess them regarding any Deprivation of

Liberty Safeguards. Each organization should have a process in place as part of hospital governance to protect vulnerable adults.

Alternatives to restraint

Any reversible cause to the agitation (such as a blocked urinary catheter or pain that needs relieving) should be treated first, before considering the use of chemical restraint – these patients may not have delirium.

Experienced and committed clinicians (doctors, nurses and others), given time and resources, can often manage an agitated cognitively impaired individual with the minimal use of restraints. It has been demonstrated that the use of physical restraints can be reduced without an increase in the use of antipsychotic drugs by educating and supporting staff. This requires constant supervision of patients and a calm consistent environment. Lipowski wrote: 'the patient is best cared for in a quiet, well-lighted room with a dimmed light at night. Staff have to use their judgment in adjusting the patient's environment according to his or her individual needs. If continuous nursing care cannot be provided and the patient is markedly disturbed, special attendants should be ordered to stay with him or her around the clock.'

Key points

- Delirious patients generally lack capacity.
- Restraints can be physical or chemical.

- Restraint can ethically be used on patients who lack capacity when needed to treat or prevent a life-threatening medical condition, assuming an advance directive is not in place.
- Restraints should always be the minimum needed and applied for the shortest possible duration. Their use should be documented.
- A patient is deprived of liberty if they are restrained physically or chemically to control behaviour rather than to enable treatment. This requires authorization.

FURTHER READING

Alzheimer's Society website with information on mental capacity issues. www.alzheimers.org.uk.

Royal College of Nursing (UK). *Let's Talk about Restraint.* London, Royal College of Nursing, 2008. www.rcn.org.uk/_data/assets/pdf_file/0007/157723/0003208.pdf.

UK Department of Health website, MCA guidance includes information on Deprivation of Liberty Safeguards. www.dh.gov.uk/en/SocialCare/Deliveringadultsocialcare/MentalCapacity/index.htm.

US hospital governance website. www.jointcommission.org/.

Chapter 11

End-of-life care

Introduction

In palliative care, delirium may be referred to as cognitive failure, terminal restlessness or terminal agitation. At least, the terminology is inconsistent in both palliative and critical care! It is sad that these names imply that delirium is an inevitable part of the dying process. Delirium episodes in palliative care are potentially reversible in up to 50% of cases.

It is estimated that one in five Americans die in US intensive care units. Patients are admitted to ICU suffering from acute episodes of chronic illnesses, and patients with advanced incurable diseases are brought in to manage consequences of treatment or progression of disease. The terminal stage of illness is sometimes only recognized after admission. Previously fit patients can succumb to the complications of acute illness, developing irreversible multiple organ failure.

Delirium is distressing for patients and caregivers, even more when it happens at the end of a life. The attention deficits impede communication with families and hinder participation in treatment decisions, counselling and symptom assessment.

Clarity of cognitive function before dying is a precious gift to patients, caregivers and relatives. In end-of-life care, clinicians have to ensure aggressive detection and management of delirium while addressing other treatment needs such as pain relief and sedation.

End-of-life care with reversible delirium

In a landmark study, Lawlor *et al.* prospectively studied 113 patients with advanced cancer admitted to an acute palliative care unit. Delirium was present in 44 patients on admission and 27 developed delirium during their stay, 20 patients had more than one episode. Of all episodes, 49% were reversible, even when accounting for terminal delirium (just before death) that was present in 88% of the 52 patients who died in hospital.

Reversibility was more common when the delirium was precipitated primarily by the use of psychoactive drugs, opioids and non-opioids, with or without dehydration. Reversibility was achieved by changing or reducing the dose of opioid drugs, discontinuing all unnecessary psychoactive medication, or simply by hydrating the patient.

Interestingly, delirium was more likely to be reversible when appearing after admission. Non-reversibility was associated with hypoxic encephalopathy and infections, as shown in other studies where non-reversibility was associated with increased organ failure.

A framework can easily be set in place to manage delirium in the terminally ill patient admitted to critical care, as suggested in Table 11.1.

Table 11.1 Framework for end-of-life ICU delirium

All or none of these measures may be appropriate for an individual patient.

- Environment: Nurse in a side room for optimal stimulation, noise and light levels.
- Medical restraints: Remove ECG leads, oximeter probes, arterial line, remove all but one peripheral intravenous cannula or CVP line if in place, loosen bedclothes.
- Dehydration: If death not imminent (up to 24–48 hours) use intravenous rehydration.
- Pain: Use opioids: start, rotate or change dose.
- Review need for drugs with anticholinergic properties (ranitidine, digoxin, furosemide).
- Hypoxia: Use high flow oxygen where respiratory support discontinued.
- Parenteral nutrition: Stop parenteral nutrition for 24 hours and review.
- Constipation: Start or change bowel regimen.
- Music: Familiar light music.
- Depression: Start/change antidepressant.
- Antipsychotics: Persist with appropriate antipsychotic therapy, prescribe regularly.

When to call in the experts?

Multiple interventions to combat symptoms in terminally ill patients might be a required step (Figure 11.1).

A palliative care team in a cancer centre in Houston, USA, reported their experience of 88 ICU referrals for uncontrolled symptom distress, family distress and end-of-life care. Half of patients were on a ventilator. All patients had advanced cancer, three quarters with metastatic disease. The team diagnosed delirium in the majority of patients (71 of the 88) and prescribed an antipsychotic (or a change in antipsychotic). They also applied other measures including a change in

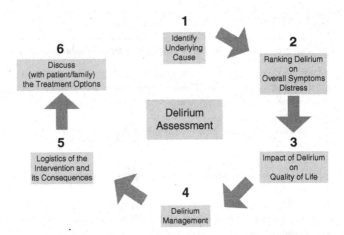

Figure 11.1 Delirium assessment in palliative care. Reprinted from *Clinics in Geriatric Medicine*, Vol. 21, Issue 1, Yennurajalingam *et al*. Pain and terminal delirium research in the elderly, Copyright 2005, pp. 93–119, with permission from Elsevier.

opioids, discontinuing benzodiazepines and anticholinergic drugs, and highlighted depression and constipation. Ventilatory support was withdrawn in all ventilated patients and high flow oxygen masks used if necessary. Delirium improved in 21 patients, and 20 patients were discharged alive; 9 discharged home with hospice services and 4 home with outpatient follow-up. Six patients underwent palliative sedation because of either uncontrolled agitation (three patients) or uncontrolled dyspnoea following withdrawal of ventilatory support (three patients).

This team believe in aggressive symptom management, especially for agitation, to decrease distress in patients,

Table 11.2 Physical and psychological symptoms after palliative care team consultation

	No. of patients (%)		
Symptoms	Symptom improvement/ symptom present	Symptoms unchanged	Symptoms worse
Pain	67/74 (90)	7 (10)	
Fatigue	34/84 (40)	48 (57)	2 (2)
Nausea	30/33 (91)	2 (6)	1 (1)
Drowsiness	27/69 (39)	31 (45)	11 (16)
Depression	19/40 (48)	21 (52)	
Anxiety	51/57 (89)	6 (11)	
Appetite	13/67 (19)	54 (81)	
Dyspnea	60/67 (90)	7 (10)	
Sleep	33/61 (54)	28 (46)	
Constipation	44/53 (83)	4 (7)	
Delirium	31/71 (44)	25 (35)	

Delgado-Guay *et al*. Symptom distress, interventions and outcomes of intensive care unit patients referred to a palliative care consult team. *Cancer* 2009; 115: 437–45. Reprinted with permission of John Wiley and Sons.

families and friends. These examples demonstrate that managing delirium in this way in this group of patients can lead to significant improvements in individual care.

Distress and delirium

Delirium is a cause of distress amongst patients, carers and clinicians. It is all the more poignant when a patient is dying. This distress has been quantified by interviews to record the recalled frequency of delirium symptoms (disorientation to time or place, visual, auditory or tactile hallucinations, delusional thoughts and psychomotor agitation) and self-reported emotional distress on a scale of 0 to 4 where 4 is extremely distressed (Figure 11.2).

This distress can be a major cause of tension between the staff and the family. This is particularly the case when the family believe that the patient's agitation is due to pain rather than as a result of delirium. Large doses of morphine can cause opioid induced delirium making the situation worse. Breitbart describes a 'double bereavement' where relatives grieve the

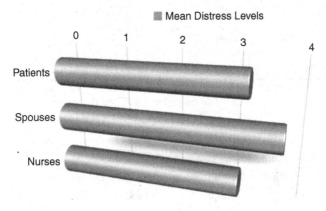

Figure 11.2. Mean distress levels for patients, spouses/caregivers, and nurses as rated on a 0–4 numerical rating scale. Reprinted from Breitbart *et al.* The delirium experience: delirium recall and delirium-related distress in hospitalized patients with cancer, their spouses/caregivers, and their nurses. *Psychosomatics* 2002; 43: 183–94. Copyright 2002, American Psychiatric Association.

loss of meaningful connection with the loved one as a result of the delirium and then grieve again when the patient dies.

The distress as remembered by the patient can be present whether the delirium is hyper- or hypoactive. One patient recorded – echoing a character in the film The Sixth Sense – that he saw dead people. The relatives are more distressed by the obvious loss of brain function and agitation.

The distress of the healthcare professional is reflected in a retrospective study analysing doses of neuroleptic use by delirium subtype. The doses of neuroleptics used were generally low, appeared ineffective in preventing delirium recall and did not correlate with delirium recall or distress the patients and families felt. The doses did increase as the nurse's distress increased with patient symptoms such as disorientation, delusions and agitation. It increased as the palliative care doctor recorded distress with the patient suffering hallucinations and agitation.

It appears inevitable that as little is known about the right dose and timing of neuroleptic drugs in delirium clinicians prescribe them according to what they see and feel rather than what the patient may actually need.

The importance of documentation

Communication with family and other relatives is always essential when patients develop delirium. Clinicians need to actively guide patients and families through the course and treatment of delirium. The clinician should explain how common it is, its relation to the illness rather than due to 'madness' or developed dementia.

Great consideration should be given to relatives expressing concerns about the delirious status of a patient. The concerns of all healthcare workers involved in the patient's management should be listened to.

A 72-year-old man with lung cancer and metastases to the left adrenal gland and left parietal lobe of his brain was admitted to a palliative care unit with increasing abdominal pain. He had been started on a combination of hydrocodone and acetaminophen 2 days earlier. On admission he was delirious, drowsy and agitated, with systemic hypertension. Most of his medical history was given by his wife. He was treated with haloperidol, which was not effective, and olanzapine was added. His pain was managed with intravenous morphine. The diagnosis of constipation was made and he was treated appropriately – opening his bowels lessened his pain, but the patient still had episodes of confusion. Clinicians thought he may have 'terminal delirium'.

At this stage, a more detailed and comprehensive history was taken from his wife and revealed he had been using a CPAP mask at night for obstructive sleep apnoea, but stopped using it 6 months before this admission. He was commenced on CPAP and his delirium improved rapidly, and resolved. Pain killers and antipsychotic medications were reduced and he remained cognitively intact and comfortable for a further 4 weeks.

This patient's delirium was caused by respiratory failure resulting from the opioids required for pain relief.

(Adapted from Reddy *et al.* [13].)

This emphasises that terminal delirium is a diagnosis of exclusion.

Clinicians should acknowledge that they know delirium is distressing to witness and explain the treatments that will be given to try and control the symptoms. Side effects of the treatments, including sedation, should be explained. Finally, relatives should be told that delirium is more common at the end of life so they can be prepared for the death of their loved one while delirium has not improved. Our ideal goal 'is a patient who is comfortable, not in pain, awake, alert, calm, cognitively intact, and able to communicate coherently with family and staff ' but 'When delirium is part of the dying process the goal may shift to providing comfort through the judicious use of sedatives, even at the expense of alertness.' (Adapted from Breitbart and Alici [11].)

Palliative sedation

When patients at the end of their lives are suffering refractory and intolerable symptoms, palliative sedation provides a last resort when other options have failed. It is usually continuous and deep although initially doses may be small enough to maintain a patient's ability to communicate periodically. There is an intense and ongoing discussion on the definition, indication and frequency of palliative sedation. The European Association for Palliative Care have put forward a recommended framework for the use of sedation in palliative care.

Palliative sedation is not indicated to control or treat delirium. Put simply, it means to start sedative and opioid infusions in a patient specifically with the aim of reducing consciousness until the patient dies. This is different from starting a propofol infusion to manage agitated delirium in the short term.

Intolerable suffering is at the heart of any decision to use palliative sedation, in other words, a symptom or state the patient or patient proxy does not wish to endure. Frequently in palliative care units, it is used to manage patients suffering delirium that is unresponsive to haloperidol. Decisions regarding hydration and nutrition are considered separately and are based on weighing up the relative benefit versus harm. The ethics related to palliative sedation is a veritable minefield and is beyond the scope of this book.

In some ICUs, the palliative care team will be consulted if a patient is suffering but not imminently dying, particularly if the patient is not already on sedative or opioid infusions. Readers interested in this subject can refer to the European Association for Palliative Care website.

ICU clinicians are often faced with having to withdraw active support from a patient who is dying despite maximal haemodynamic and respiratory support. In these patients sedative and opioid infusions are often already in place to maintain comfort and are generally continued until death.

Key points

- Delirium is common in the terminally ill patient.
- Up to 50% of delirium episodes are potentially reversible by changing analgesic drugs, modifying the doses of drugs, or ensuring proper hydration.

- The management of delirium must be balanced with the aim of an overall reduction in suffering.
- Families and friends find delirium in patients at the end of life particularly distressing.

FURTHER READING

Breitbart W and Alici Y. Agitation and delirium at the end of life "we couldn't manage him". *Journal of the American Medical Association* 2008; 300: 2898–910.

Caraceni A and Grassi L. *Delirium: Acute Confusional States in Palliative Medicine*, 2nd edn. New York, Oxford University Press, 2011.

Cherny NI, Radbruch L; The Board of the European Association for Palliative Care. European Association for Palliative Care (EAPC) recommended framework for the use of sedation in palliative care. *Palliative Medicine* 2009; 23(7): 581–93. www.eapcnet.org/projects/Sedation.html.

US National Cancer Institute. *Cognitive Disorders and Delirium PDQ summary.* www.cancer.gov/cancertopics/pdq/ supportivecare/delirium/HealthProfessional.

Chapter 12

What is the future?

The facts

As discussed in Chapter 1, Engel and Romano bemoaned in 1959 that the clinician fails to recognize delirium and is more concerned to 'protect the functional integrity of the heart, liver and kidneys of his patient but has not learnt to have similar regard for the functional integrity of the brain'.

What we do know

Delirium in ICU is a condition that develops overall in approximately one in three patients, and in two of three patients needing mechanical ventilation.

ICU delirium is frequently missed and its duration is linked to an increasing risk of mortality. It is associated with significantly worse outcomes including long-term cognitive impairment.

Some cases are preventable.

What we don't know

Many things. . . we have more questions than answers and probably will have for some time to come. Some questions are listed in Table 12.1.

Table 12.1 Unanswered questions about delirium in critical care

How many cases of delirium are preventable?

Will treating delirium definitely improve patient outcomes?

Will preventing delirium improve patient outcomes?

Do any antipsychotics treat the symptoms or the cause of delirium?

Do any antipsychotics work in hypoactive delirium?

What about delirium in children?

What are the changes in the brain in delirium?

Is there a relation between delirium and long-term cognitive impairment?

What are the risk factors?

Does delirium worsen sepsis?

How important is genetics in delirium?

Is delirium an early indicator of dementia?

Is sedation-inducing inattention delirium?

How significant is subsyndromal delirium?

Is sleep deprivation a cause or result of delirium?

Do alpha agonists prevent or treat delirium?

Would an anti-inflammatory intervention modify delirium?

Can persistent delirium be treated?

Is there a reliable biomarker for delirium?

Should we ban the use of physical restraints?

Should we never use benzodiazepines again in ICU?

How can we implement routine ICU delirium monitoring?

Education

Screening for delirium should be a routine fact of ICU life, just like measuring urine output! The brain is the most important organ in the body. It is the one organ everyone wants intact on discharge. Education is required to ensure this happens, and education takes time.

The fact that this has not been taken into account before does not make it unimportant now. Consider how important the immune system is in sepsis and that the intact brain modulates the immune system. As we learn more we'll put more pieces together – this is the beginning.

Within many critical care units, there is a resistance to implementing delirium screening. Several explanations are given and include practical difficulties (or pragmatism as some may call it) and a scientifico-clinical scepticism. Change implementation of any kind is always difficult. This is another demand on very busy nurses or doctors, and nurses will probably abandon a screening task if it results in no action. The connection between detection and treatment must be understood. The impact of delirium on outcome must be known.

The brain is the organ of consciousness, arousal and cognition. Delirium is a failure of cognition, an organ failure. And up to 65% of critically ill patients in the UK (most are ventilated) develop delirium and some will suffer adverse outcomes... so single organ failure suddenly becomes a rarity!

The evidence gathered to date would strongly indicate that delirium is in itself a danger to our patients but more studies are needed. Occurrence of delirium is a sign of a change in patient status and may be the first or only sign. It may indicate a new infection, an adverse response to a drug or a level of hypoxia that will result in long-term cognitive impairment. It is a clinical event that needs to be actively managed.

Screening is a unique interaction with the critically ill patient, which requires a cognitive response. Patients and loved ones are concerned about the integrity of their brains. Even in the patient who is not delirious, having a clinician establishing even a brief exchange, a two-way rather than one-way interaction, is reassuring.

Outside critical care, the routine screening for delirium in high-risk patients is considered good practice.

Research priorities

Current research priorities include laboratory work to determine the pathophysiology of this complex multifactorial syndrome. Knowing for sure whether antipsychotics work to reverse delirium or just on the symptoms will end a lot of discussion between delirium experts.

Sophisticated neuroimaging studies may help understand specific anatomical, molecular and functional features of central nervous system decline. Longitudinal studies can examine neuroimaging changes of longer-term cognitive decline.

There are increasing numbers of published clinical observational studies establishing the extent and degree of the problem in different patient populations. These can only achieve so much regarding changing clinical practice to improve patients' experience and outcomes.

The results of intervention studies into preventing or treating delirium are awaited, whether they look at non-pharmacological or pharmacological interventions to prevent or treat the delirium. Work is needed to establish whether there are any benefits in treating patients.

Pharmacological treatment of delirium

Antipsychotics and in particular haloperidol are the first-line treatment used for delirium. Recent evidence suggests that haloperidol is useful to decrease agitation but does not modify delirium. It is unknown whether this applies to all populations, sicker or healthier patients. It is unknown whether atypical antipsychotics are effective in critically ill patients.

Evaluation of new agents is promising, but more is needed. Prospective studies, of various compounds head to head, are definitely required.

Sedation techniques

Studies are needed to balance the risks and benefits of analgesic and sedative drugs in relation to delirium. Studies on the impact of sedation protocols on the duration of ventilation abound, but only a few look at the impact on delirium.

Publicizing delirium: education!

The European Delirium Association was set up in 2006 and the American Delirium Society followed in 2009. Researchers and practitioners from all over the world join efforts to cover delirium research, clinical practice and promotion of better care. Associations and Societies enable collaboration between centres nationally and internationally and include a broad range of practices: from delirium in the community to hospital settings, and from the paediatric patient to the extremely elderly. Similar organizations are set up in other parts of the world, such as Australia.

Key point

Delirium in critical care is a developing field – Watch this space!

FURTHER READING

www.europeandeliriumassociation.com.

http://www.americandeliriumsociety.org.

http://www.youtube.com/user/IntensiveCareAu?
    feature=watch.

SELECTED REFERENCES

1. Lipowski ZJ. *Delirium: Acute Confusional States*. New York, Oxford University Press, 1990.
2. Inouye SK *et al*. Nurse recognition of delirium and its symptoms: comparison of nurse and researcher ratings. *Archives of Internal Medicine* 2001; 161: 2467–73.
3. van Eijk MM *et al*. Comparison of delirium assessment tools in a mixed intensive care unit. *Critical Care Medicine* 2009; 37: 1881–5.
4. Spronk PE *et al*. Occurrence of delirium is severely underestimated in the ICU during daily care. *Intensive Care Medicine* 2009; 35: 1276–80.
5. Grassi L *et al*. Depression or hypoactive delirium? A report of ciprofloxacin-induced mental disorder in a patient with chronic obstructive pulmonary disease. *Psychotherapy and Psychosomatics* 2001; 70: 58–9.
6. Dunn WF *et al*. Iatrogenic delirium and coma: a near miss. *Chest* 2008; 133: 1217–20.
7. Spiller JA and Keen JC. Hypoactive delirium: assessing the extent of the problem for inpatient specialist palliative care. *Palliative Medicine* 2006; 20: 17–23.

8. Angles EM *et al*. Risk factors for delirium after major trauma. *American Journal of Surgery* 2008; 196: 864–70.

9. Luetz A *et al*. Different assessment tools for intensive care unit delirium: which score to use. *Critical Care Medicine* 2010; 38: 409–18.

10. Coyle N *et al*. Delirium as a contributing factor to "crescendo" pain: three case reports. *Journal of Pain and Symptom Management* 1994; 9: 44–7.

11. Breitbart W and Alici Y. Agitation and delirium at the end of life: "we couldn't manage him". *Journal of the American Medical Association* 2008; 300: 2898–910.

12. Annas GJ. The last resort – the use of physical restraints in medical emergencies. *New England Journal of Medicine* 1999; 341: 1408–12.

13. Reddy S *et al*. Opioids masquerading as delirium in a patient with cancer pain and obstructive sleep apnea. *Journal of Palliative Medicine* 2008; 11: 1043–5.

INDEX

Printed in the United States
By Bookmasters